THE THEORY AND PRACTICE OF 3D PET

Developments in Nuclear Medicine

VOLUME 32

Series Editor: Peter H. Cox

The Theory and Practice of 3D PET

edited by

BERNARD BENDRIEM

Service Hospitalier Frédéric Joliot,
Orsay, France

and

DAVID W. TOWNSEND

University of Pittsburgh,
Pittsburgh, PA, U.S.A.

SPRINGER-SCIENCE+BUSINESS MEDIA, B.V.

A C.I.P. Catalogue record for this book is available from the Library of Congress.

ISBN 978-90-481-5040-3 ISBN 978-94-017-3475-2 (eBook)
DOI 10.1007/978-94-017-3475-2

This printing is a digital duplication of the original edition.

Second Printing 2003

CONTENTS

Foreword *by Terry Jones* vii
Preface xiii
List of Contributors xv

1. INTRODUCTION TO 3D PET 1
D.W. Townsend and B. Bendriem

Introduction 1
Reconstruction algorithms 5
Reconstruction times 5
Scatter correction 6
Normalization 6
Attenuation correction 6
Summary 7
References 7

2. DATA ACQUISITION AND IMAGE RECONSTRUCTION FOR 3D PET 11
M. Defrise and P.E. Kinahan

3D PET Data Acquisition 11
Review of 2D image reconstruction 22
Image Reconstruction for 3D PET 31
Alternative 3D Reconstruction Methods 42
Noise 47
References 50

3. QUANTITATIVE PROCEDURES IN 3D PET 55
D.L. Bailey, *with contributions from:*
M-C. Gilardi, S. Grootoonk, P.E. Kinahan, C. Nahmias,
J. Ollinger, D.W. Townsend, R. Trébossen, and M. Zito

Introduction 55
Scatter in 3D PET Measurements 56
Assessing the Accuracy of Scatter Correction (DLB, MCG, MZ) 61
Scatter Correction (DLB, SG, JO, RT) 64
Scatter from outside the field-of-view 84
Normalisation Methods for 3D PET (DB, PEK, DWT) 86
Attenuation Correction for 3D PET (DLB, CN) 98
Calibration in 3D PET 100
References 101

4. VOLUME IMAGING TOMOGRAPHS 111
D. W. Townsend, R. A. Isoardi and B. Bendriem

Introduction 111
Performance Characteristics 112
Three Dimenional Data Sets 124
Three-Dimensional Reconstruction 127
Conclusion 129
References 130

5. APPLICATIONS OF 3D PET 133
K. Wienhard, *with contributions from*:
DL Bailey, A Bol, DJ Brooks, T Bruckbauer, PD Cutler L Eriksson, L Farde, S Grootoonk, WD Heiss, T Jones, K Herholz, M Ingvar, C Michel, MP Miller, PK Morrish, U Pietrzyk, JS Rakshi, P Remy, A Thiel, R. Trébossen, and AG De Volder

Introduction 133
Experience of 3D PET at the Karolinska Hospital (LE, LF, MI) 134
Performing activation studies with 3D PET (SG) 136
Optimization of the [^{18}F]FDG protocol for clinical cerebral studies in 3D PET (PR, RT) 141
Contribution of 3D acquisition in pediatric neurology (AGV, AB, CM) 144
Clinical applications of 3D PET in brain tumors (KH, AT, TB, UP, WDH) 148
3D ^{18}F-Fluorodopa PET: improved kinetics and discrimination in Parkinson's disease (DLB, DJB, TJ, MPM, PKM, JSR) 150
Whole-body imaging in 3D (DC) 154
References 162

FOREWORD

Future Prospects for 3D PET

In writing a Foreword to this monograph, I was asked to focus on the future prospects for 3D PET. This is a logical perspective since without a future there is little point in detailing the methodology and describing how it can be implemented and improved.

Why 3D PET?

Positron Emission Tomography is the most sensitive means for imaging trace levels of molecules *in vivo*. Hence a starting point of why 3D clearly is to reinforce this strength by fully exploiting the technology of electronic collimation offered through coincidence counting.

Scientific research tends to stem from technology thrusts. Hence advances in technology are often to be founded within the research applications where in general, increases in sensitivity and specificity are the drive for making more precise scientific observations. Therefore, in the first instance, it is appropriate to identify the stimulus for using 3D PET within the research community. Here the emphasis is on obtaining new information on human disease and its treatment.

At a mundane, yet important, level when administering radioactivity to subjects, volunteering for a PET research procedure, be they normal subjects or patients, a prime consideration is to minimise radiation exposure. There is a limit to how much radiation exposure can be ethically administered for research procedures which offer no benefit to the subjects being studied. Indeed, this limit is ever decreasing in the light of recommendations being developed by the International Commission for Radiological Protection to reduce doses. A principal directive is that radiation doses should be kept to the minimum necessary for the procedure. Here the emphasis must be to maximise the signal per unit of absorbed radiation dose. The specific stimuli for this are:

- To record PET scan kinetic data so that it is, on statistical grounds, possible to implement a voxel by voxel analysis to produce functional parametric images which retain the inherent spatial resolution of the tomograph.

- To accurately measure low concentrations of tracer binding sites, e.g. ligand-receptor interactions which are of pharmacological importance and may be perturbed in disease states. Examples of these are the dopaminergic receptors in the cerebral cortex which reside at one tenth of the level of those in the striatum of the brain. Sub-types of such receptors are becoming of increasing importance despite their expression being secondary to the main receptor sub-type.

- Kinetic analysis can be used to separate out specific from non-specific binding including the accumulation of radiolabelled metabolites. Accurate delineation of the shape of the kinetic time courses offers the chance of interpreting signal recorded with less than perfect radioligands and radiotracers which are associated with significant background levels in the tissue of interest.

- To enable repeat studies to be undertaken in order to investigate the functional time course of a disease and its response to physiological challenges and treatment effects.

- To accurately follow the kinetics of rapidly decaying tracer and ensure the latter time data, which is important for delineating the kinetics, does not compromise the precision of the parametric images. The use of ^{11}C-labelled tracers and ligands are such an example. During a one to two hour study encompassing 6-8 half-lives of this radionuclide, it is important to avoid statistically compromising the later stage data. As an additional point, it is worth stressing that with respect to recording the maximum signal per unit of radiation absorbed dose, a goal is to continuously collect data during the time the tracer is effectively present in the body. This is analogous to radiological procedures where exposure is confined to the time of the data collection. In this respect, ^{11}C is attractive since 1-2 hour duration studies are feasible with the subject remaining within the tomograph. In addition to recording good statistical data at the end of the time course of a study, it is worth emphasising that the device used needs to be linear in its response over the whole procedure. Losses in effective counts due to deadtime and randoms registration need to be minimised especially at the initial high count rate stage when the tracer is administered.

- To enhance the discovery of new, specific radioligands, which focus on measuring low concentrations of binding sites. This is based on the need to find increasingly high affinity tracer molecules. Inevitably this leads to the need to increase the specific activity of the formulated tracer in order to minimise blockade of the binding site with the accompanying cold compound. This limits how much tracer can be administered without perturbing the recorded signal and represents another stimulus for minimising administered doses (hot unlabelled and labelled compound) and yet still retain statistically-significant tomographic data. Not all radiotracer studies are confined to a few hours study since sequestration may take many hours or days including the clearance of non-specific background levels. This demands the use of longer-lived, ^{18}F or even such radionuclides as ^{124}I with its 4.1 day half-life. Clearly under radiation dose restrictions, sensitivity becomes a major issue if the accuracy of such recorded data is not to be compromised.

Applications of 3D PET

Having described the broad brush of why sensitivity is such an important issue, it is worth itemising areas where this sensitivity is finding a research outlet. The justification for clinical research, as opposed to basic experimental biological studies, rests primarily on the need to study human disease states where suitable models do not exist. High in this justification is the psychiatric area, which includes studies in schizophrenia, depression, anxiety and addiction. These are paralleled with studies to investigate cognition including memory in normal subjects in order to identify perturbations in disease. This area is being embraced through PET blood flow activation studies now being contributed to by fMRI. However, the underlying neurochemical processes in such cerebral functions is only now being addressed with PET. Neurological diseases encompassing dementia, stroke recovery and movement disorders still necessitate human investigations. In cancer, while experimental animal tumours are extensively studied, the peculiarities of the human cancers still need to be investigated to address differences between experimental and clinical conditions.

The evolution of such base-line clinical research would be to use PET in drug discovery and development. Here, a central focus, and one that dominates the pharmaceutical industry, is to derive the "proof of principle" of the action and efficacy of a new therapy. As drug development becomes increasingly competitive and expensive, early "proof of principle" is essential in decisions to proceed with development. It also provides scientific feedback to discovery teams of medicinal chemists, chemo informatics, drug modellers, pharmacologists etc. PET, through its specificity and sensitivity offers "proof of principle" how the binding site of interest, which is to be perturbed by the novel therapy, is expressed *in vivo* and that the drug being developed actually modifies this expression. Novel information is further available through tissue pharmacokinetics and tissue dosimetry of the radiolabelled drug itself. This is important as 50% of drugs that fail in development do so for pharmacokinetic reasons. Additional "proof of principle" comes from using PET to study pharmacodynamic effects of the drug, namely changes in specific functional activity of the tissue, e.g. reduced metabolism or proliferative activity of a tumour. This whole area can be considered as one of translation from basic biology and drug discovery programmes to the clinic. When fully mobilised this will bring a huge intellectual property base which promises to enhance clinical research activities using PET.

In order to facilitate and enhance this translation, consideration is now focusing on the PET scanning of experimental laboratory animal models used by biologists and drug discoverers in development of therapeutic strategies. Indeed, some pharmaceutical companies will not enter a disease area unless they have suitable laboratory animal model of the pathology in question. Here the use of transgenic animals with their genetic delineation which model the disease state is dominant. Since such transgenics are produced principally in the laboratory mouse, the challenge to PET is to be able to record accurate PET data in such small *in vivo* structures. The case for increased sensitivity as itemised for human studies, apart from radiation doses, comes to bear with the heightened challenge of the small physical scale for which it is required. Clearly the thrust is to recover the maximum spatial resolution achievable. This points to maximum sensitivity, especially as there are limits to the amount of cold compound which can be administered, and hence the stimulation for 3D data recording.

Thought needs to be given to the role 3D PET in the clinical diagnostic area. Currently this is dominated by staging in oncology where the emphasis is on using ^{18}FDG to delineate secondary disease in mainly adult patients. Clearly radiation absorbed dose consideration is of less importance in this clinical population. A possible development would be to use ^{124}I-labelled antibodies with a view to employing more specific markers of neoplasia especially where the focus is to delineate interstitial disease near to the primary lesion. This would have implications, for example, in accurately delineating radiotherapy fields and changes therein during a course of fractionation. ^{18}FDG is being used to help work up young epileptic patients prior to surgery and here high sensitivity 3D PET should be the technology of choice.

In the future, psychiatric research with PET could begin to uncover characteristic receptor binding and neurotransmitter pathways in, for example, schizophrenia using ^{18}F-L-dopa and ^{18}F-metatyrosine. This could migrate into the diagnostic area where young teenage patients presenting for the first time may need to have their neurochemistry characterised prior to selecting the optimal neuroleptic. Clearly high sensitivity 3D scanning of tracers of neurotransmission which have relatively poor brain uptake would again be the technology of choice.

Development of 3D PET

Having defined the case for implementing and developing 3D PET, it is now appropriate to examine how it should evolve from the present state. In the first instance, concern needs to be focused on the optimal use of current 3D technology. It will be clear from the following chapters that in the current use of bismuth germanate (BGO) and sodium iodide (NaI) involving integral crystal designs, dead time and randoms registration impose a significant loss of effective counts at high activity. Hence the first consideration is to reduce the amount of radioactivity administered so that these losses are minimised. This occurred when 3D PET was first introduced for brain activation studies using $H_2^{15}O$. Statistical losses resulting from subtraction of random coincidences suggest the implementation of spatial and temporal averaging of the randoms to help reduce this source of noise. Further work is required with respect to scatter correction in body structures and statistically uncompromising transmission data is needed. Here segmentation of organ outlines and the assigning of fixed attenuation factors need to be perfected, especially in the body. The use of iterative reconstruction continues to show promise in PET. Here the challenge is to capitalise upon the efficiency of the 3D and implement iterative reconstructions for multiple frame 3D kinetic data. Given the improved statistics resulting from 3D, the implementation of iterative reconstruction which builds in a deconvolution of the resolution response function of the scanner represents an appreciable, and yet achievable, challenge.

A major hurdle is the use of 3D for body studies. The large contribution from out of the "coincidence field of view" activity imposes dead time and random effects which need careful strategies to minimise loss of effective counts. High sensitivity 3D PET encourages strategies to maximise the temporal resolution within the data set. This indicates the use of list mode data collection which is also cost effective in data storage. The challenge here is to collect and reconstruct such data sets in a routine way. List mode offers the optimal way to effect physiological gating studies and also a data storage efficient means for recording the total energy spectrum for each coincidence event. The stimulus for this is to effect, especially for the body, accurate scatter correction routines based upon the information contained within the energy spectrum.

While current 3D PET tomographs have a great deal of scope for application with respect to optimum data collection and processing, it is clear that the introduction of scintillation crystals with faster rise and decay times and with increased emission of light would greatly enhance the performance and dynamic range of 3D PET. The new scintillator, lutetium oxyorthosilicate (LSO) promises to offer a significant advantage in this area, especially for body studies with their high dead time and randoms registration. To fully exploit the advantage of 3D, small ring diameter tomographs are being considered which maximise the solid angle and minimise the amount and hence cost of detector material. Here the challenge is to record the depth of interaction in the detectors in order to overcome the parallax problem resulting from such broad solid angles. The first LSO-based 3D-only tomograph with depth of interaction is currently being developed and is due to be delivered to the Cologne PET centre in 1998 and we await with interest the increased signal that this development promises to provide.

London, March 1998

Terry Jones
MRC Cyclotron Unit
Hammersmith Hospital
London, UK.

PREFACE

Since the early nineteen-fifties, Positron Emission Tomography (PET) has been recognized as an intrinsically three-dimensional (3D) imaging technique. However, only in recent years has significant effort been devoted to the development of methodology for the acquisition and reconstruction of PET data in 3D. The majority of this work has appeared in diverse scientific journals and to date, no attempt has been made to collect these important developments into a single volume. Since the application of 3D methodology has been receiving increasing attention at many PET centres, this monograph is an attempt to fill that gap and provide a state-of-the-art review, covering 3D reconstruction methods, quantitative procedures, current tomograph performance, and clinical and research applications.

The monograph aims to provide the PET researcher with the historical background and introduction to the concepts of 3D PET (Chapter 1), a detailed treatment of the theory of 3D reconstruction algorithms (Chapter 2), and a complete description of the correction procedures required to achieve fully quantitative physiological measurements from data acquired in 3D (Chapter 3). The physical performance characteristics of volume imaging tomographs are described and compared with their standard 2D operation (Chapter 4), and finally contributions from a number of different PET centres describing both clinical and research applications for which 3D plays an essential role are collected in Chapter 5. In all chapters, the subject matter is treated in depth and should appeal equally to the physicist or engineer who wishes to implement the methodology, and to PET investigators with experience in 2D PET who wish to familiarize themselves with the concepts and advantages of 3D, and to be made aware of the pitfalls. The monograph summarizes the current status of the methodology, and offers answers to questions that investigators may ask when planning their 3D studies.

The chapters in this monograph are written by leading scientists and physicians who have played key roles in establishing 3D PET as a practical methodology. The monograph has been prepared with the support of the EEC Concerted Action on PET Investigations of Cellular Regeneration and Degeneration, under the coordination of the Instrumentation Task Group. It provides a comprehensive overview of 3D PET which should appeal to scientists, engineers and clinical researchers active in the field.

Bernard Bendriem
David W. Townsend   March 1998

LIST OF CONTRIBUTORS

D.L. Bailey
MRC Cyclotron Unit
Hammersmith Hospital
Ducane Rd, London W12 0NN, UK

A. Bol
PET Laboratory
Université Catholique de Louvain
Louvain-la-Neuve, 1348 Belgium

B. Bendriem
Service Hospitalier Frédéric Joliot
DSV/DRM-CEA
4 Place du Général Leclerc
91406 Orsay, France

D.J. Brooks
MRC Cyclotron Unit
Hammersmith Hospital
Ducane Rd, London W12 0NN, UK

T. Bruckbauer
CTI PET Systems
810, Innovation Drive
Knoxville, TN 37932, USA

P.D. Cutler
Mallinckrodt Radiology
Box 8225, 510 S Kingshighway Blvd
St Louis, MO 63110, USA

M. Defrise
Department of Nuclear Medicine
AZ-VUB, Vrije Universiteit
Laarbeeklaan 101
Brussels B-1090, Belgium

L. Eriksson
CTI PET Systems
810, Innovation Drive
Knoxville, TN 37932, USA
and
Department of Neurophysiology
Karolinska Hospital
Stockholm, Sweden 17176

L. Farde
Department of Clinical Neuroscience
Section of Psychiatry and Psychology
Karolinska Institute
Stockholm, Sweden 17176

M-C. Gilardi
Department of Nuclear Medicine
Hospital San Raffaele
Via Olgettina 60
Milano, Italy

S. Grootoonk
Wellcome Department of Cognitive Neurology
Functional Imaging Laboratory
Queen Square
London WC1N 3BG, UK

W-D. Heiss
Max-Planck-Institut für neurologische Forschung
Gleueler Str. 50
W 5000 Köln 41, Germany

K. Herholz
Max-Planck-Institut für neurologische Forschung
Gleueler Str. 50
W 5000 Köln 41, Germany

M. Ingvar
Department of Clinical Neuroscience
Karolinska Hospital
Stockholm, Sweden 17176

R.A. Isoardi
Fundacion Escuela de Medicina Nuclear
Garibaldi 405
5500 Mendoza, Argentina
and
PET Facility, Department of Radiology
University of Pittsburgh Medical Center
Pittsburgh PA 15213, USA

T. Jones
MRC Cyclotron Unit
Hammersmith Hospital
Ducane Rd, London W12 0NN, UK

P.E. Kinahan
PET Facility, Department of Radiology
University of Pittsburgh Medical Center
Pittsburgh PA 15213, USA

C. Michel
PET Laboratory
Université Catholique de Louvain
Louvain-la-Neuve, Belgium 1348

M.P. Miller
MRC Cyclotron Unit
Hammersmith Hospital
Ducane Rd, London W12 0NN, UK

P.K. Morrish
MRC Cyclotron Unit
Hammersmith Hospital
Ducane Rd, London W12 0NN, UK

C. Nahmias
Department of Nuclear Medicine
McMaster University Medical Center
Hamilton, Ontario N2L3Z5, Canada

J. Ollinger
Neuroimaging Lab
Camp Bx 8225, 4525 Scott Ave
Washington University
St Louis, MO 63110, USA

U. Pietrzyk
Max-Planck-Institut für neurologische Forschung
Gleueler Str. 50
W 5000 Köln 41, Germany

J.S. Rakshi
MRC Cyclotron Unit
Hammersmith Hospital
Ducane Rd, London W12 0NN, UK

P. Remy
Service Hospitalier Frédéric Joliot
DSV/DRM-CEA
4 Place du Général Leclerc
91406 Orsay, France
and
CHU Mondor
94010 Creteil, France

A. Thiel
Max-Planck-Institut für neurologische Forschung
Gleueler Str. 50
W 5000 Köln 41, Germany

D.W. Townsend
PET Facility, Department of Radiology
University of Pittsburgh Medical Center
Pittsburgh PA 15213, USA

R. Trébossen
Service Hospitalier Frédéric Joliot
DSV/DRM-CEA
4 Place du Général Leclerc
91406 Orsay, France

A.G. De Volder
PET Laboratory
Université Catholique de Louvain
Louvain-la-Neuve, Belgium 1348

K. Wienhard
Max-Planck-Institut für neurologische Forschung
Gleueler Str. 50
W 5000 Köln 41, Germany

M. Zito
Ospedale Maggiore de Milano
Department of Nuclear Medicine
Via F.Sforza 35
Milano 20122, Italy

Chapter 1. INTRODUCTION TO 3D PET

David W. Townsend[1] and Bernard Bendriem[2]

[1] PET Facility, Department of Radiology, University of Pittsburgh, USA
[2] Service Hospitalier Frédéric Joliot, DSV/DRM-CEA, Orsay, France

Introduction

Positron Emission Tomography (PET) is intrinsically a three-dimensional (3D) imaging technique. Neutron-deficient isotopes may undergo nuclear decay by the emission of a positron, or positive electron, and a neutrino. A positron has the same mass, but opposite charge, to that of the electron. Depending on the specific isotope, positrons are emitted with a small amount of energy (a few MeV, maximum), which they rapidly lose by collisions with the atoms in the surrounding medium (tissue). Once the positron energy becomes sufficiently small, an encounter with a free electron in the tissue results in a matter-antimatter annihilation from which two photons emerge almost 180° opposed (fig. 1.1). The range of the positron in tissue from the point of emission to the point of annihilation with an electron may be a few millimeters, depending on the energy of emission from the nucleus. Deviation from 180° occurs when the positron-electron system has some residual momentum which must be conserved in the annihilation process. The energy of each of the photons from positron annihilation is 511 keV, equal to the rest mass of the electron or positron. The pairs of 511 keV annihilation photons are then emitted into a 4π solid angle (i.e. in 3D) without any particular preferential direction. Detection in coincidence of the pairs of photons from individual annihilations yields information on the underlying distribution of the positron-emitting tracer.

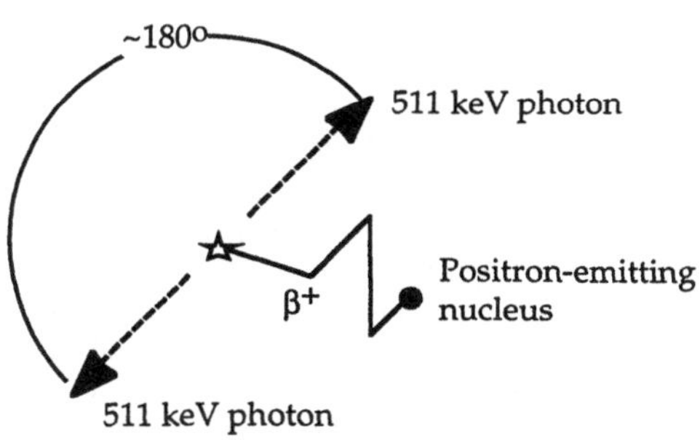

Figure 1.1 Schematic of positron emission and annihilation

B. Bendriem and D.W. Townsend (eds.) The Theory and Practice of 3D PET, 1-10.

A major importance of PET lies in the physiological nature of elements such as carbon, nitrogen and oxygen that have convenient positron-emitting isotopes. Such nuclides can be used to label natural substrates, chemically indistinguishable from their unlabeled counterpart, which participate in human metabolism. Only trace amounts of the substrates need to be administered, thus avoiding perturbation of the metabolic process that is being studied. A drawback of these physiological molecules is the short half-lives of the isotopes (2 min for ^{15}O, 10 min for ^{13}N and 20 min for ^{11}C), thus requiring a cyclotron on-site for production and allowing little time for radioactive labelling of the substrate. However, the use of short lived nuclides potentially offers more favourable dosimetry than the use of longer-lived isotopes. A fourth positron-emitting isotope, ^{18}F, is widely used to label, among other substrates, the glucose analog, deoxyglucose (DG) to form ^{18}F-labeled fluorodeoxyglucose (FDG), a tracer of glucose metabolism. With a 110 min half-life, ^{18}F is a convenient nuclide that can be produced off-site at a remote cyclotron and transported to the PET facility.

Once the tracer has been injected and allowed time to concentrate in the organ of interest, the distribution of the tracer within the organ can be recovered by collecting coincident pairs of annihilation photons. To reconstruct the distribution, two assumptions must be made: that the line along which the photons are emitted contains the location of the nucleus from which the positron originated, and that the annihilation photons are emitted 180° opposed. These assumptions are only approximately satisfied, and both the distance travelled by the positron from the point of emission and the acollinearity of the annihilation photons limit the ultimate spatial resolution attainable with the coincidence technique. Within these approximations, the integral of all photon pairs emitted along a given direction represents the sum, or line integral, of positron emitting activity lying on, or close to, this line.

In practice, the measured line integrals must be corrected for a number of background effects before reconstruction. Pairs of photons detected in coincidence but originating from two different positron annihilation events are termed random, or false, coincidences, and photons which interact and scatter in tissue before leaving the subject are either detected and assigned to an incorrect line-of-response (LOR), or are undetected and contribute to the effect of photon attenuation. Therefore, assuming that the integrals are first corrected for randoms, scatter and attenuation, as described in Chapter 3, the set of integrals having the same angular direction through the tracer distribution comprises a parallel projection of the distribution at that angle. Photon pairs are emitted along directions at random and are collected and sorted in real time into parallel projections according to their direction. The underlying tracer distribution that gives rise to these parallel projections is then reconstructed using techniques to be described in this monograph (Chapter 2).

A counting technique where individual photon pairs are collected is subject to noise arising from the statistical nature of radioactive decay and radiation detection. It is therefore important to capture as many of the photon pairs as possible during the relatively short duration of the imaging process. A number of factors limit the events that can be acquired, including the level of positron-emitting radioactivity administered, the fraction of tracer concentrating within the organ of interest, and the performance characteristics and solid-angle coverage of the PET scanner. In human studies, radioactive dose becomes an issue of limiting radiation exposure to the subject, whereas tracer uptake is related to the physiology and metabolism of the labelled substrate injected.

In the past fifteen years, extensive efforts have been devoted to improving the performance of PET scanners, and in particular, parameters such as spatial resolution, intrinsic detector efficiency and solid angle coverage. A number of prototype devices, developed at research centers in the US and Europe, introduced new concepts in PET instrumentation, which led to advances in detector technology, scanner designs and data acquisition systems. Developments in detector technology explored the use of either inorganic scintillators, such as sodium iodide [Muehllehner, 1975], bismuth germanate (BGO) [Cho and Faruhki, 1977], cesium fluoride [Allemand et al., 1980], barium fluoride [Laval et al., 1983], and gadolinium orthosilicate [Dahlbom et al., 1985], or multi-wire chambers [Townsend et al., 1987]. In the early eighties, a number of groups explored the possibility of using time-of-flight information to localize the positron annihilation. Although the timing resolution was insufficient to obtain exact localization of the annihilation event, some improvement in signal-to-noise was achieved by incorporating time-of-flight information into the reconstruction process. A tomograph exploiting time-of-flight information and based on barium fluoride was successfully developed during the eighties [Mazoyer et al., 1990].

Initially, scanner designs were based on hexagonal or circular arrays of individual crystals imaging a single transaxial slice, or dual rotating area detectors covering a large axial field of view. In an effort to improve the axial coverage of the single-slice scanners, multi-slice systems were developed by stacking individual rings or hexagonal arrays. The multi-ring configuration eventually emerged as the preferred design for commercial tomographs. A major advance in the design of multi-ring scanners occurred in the mid-eighties with the appearance of the block detector [Casey and Nutt, 1986] as a cost-effective way to couple small crystals to photomultiplier tubes (PMTs) without requiring a dedicated PMT for each crystal (fig. 1.2). Blocks of BGO cut into an array of 8 x 8 small crystals are glued to four PMTs. The cuts between the crystals are of different depths and, for each crystal, light is shared among the four PMTs in a unique way. To localize the crystal in which the incident 511 keV photon interacted, the output signals from the PMTs are compared. PET scanners covering an axial field-of-view (FOV) of 10 cm with eight rings of crystals became available in 1986, and by 1990, improved axial sampling was possible with up to sixteen detector rings covering a 10 cm axial FOV. Since the early nineties, the demand for increased axial coverage has led to the point where current commercial state-of-the-art scanners have an axial FOV of over 15 cm, sampled by up to 32 rings of detectors.

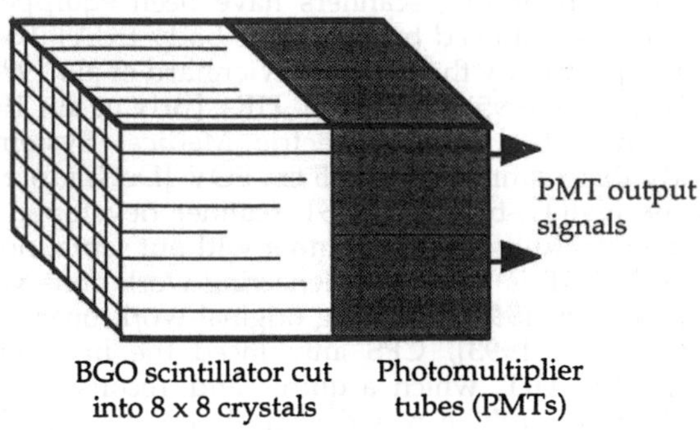

Figure 1.2 The BGO block detector [Casey and Nutt, 1986]

An important feature of the early multi-ring scanners was the presence of fixed annular septa, composed of a lead-tungsten alloy, positioned between the detector rings. The septa, although only 1-2 mm thick, project 8-10 cm from the detector face, shielding the crystals from photons emitted obliquely to the planes of the detector rings. The septa serve two purposes: first, to shield the detectors from photons which scatter out of the plane of a detector ring, and second, to limit data acquisition and reconstruction to a set of contiguous 2D planes aligned with the detector rings. Reducing scatter eliminates the need for a sophisticated scatter correction algorithm, and limiting the acquisition and reconstruction to 2D avoids the considerable complexity of a fully 3D reconstruction algorithm. These factors were essential in the mid-eighties since, at that time, neither accurate scatter correction techniques nor 3D reconstruction algorithms had been developed for multi-ring scanners.

However, the benefits of septa are offset by a significant sensitivity loss due to 2D acquisition of an intrinsically 3D emission process. In multi-ring scanners with septa, electronic collimation, which is the efficient way of imaging positron emitting tracers through the use of coincidence detection rather than physical collimation, is not fully exploited. Septa introduce physical collimation in the axial direction and limit acquisition to LORs involving crystals in the same or nearby detector rings, thus eliminating the more oblique LORs.

During the early eighties, fully 3D reconstruction algorithms were developed for PET imaging using large area wire-chamber detectors. In 1988, it was realized that the fully 3D reconstruction algorithms developed for the wire-chamber were applicable, with some modifications, to multi-ring scanners. Thus, in 1988, in a series of studies, the septa were physically removed from the ECAT 931, an eight-ring PET scanner built by CTI PET Systems (Knoxville, TN) and installed at Hammersmith Hospital in London. With the septa removed, 3D data sets were acquired for the ECAT 931 at a count rate of more than eight times higher than the count rate for a comparable study with the septa in place; the count rate in 3D includes a factor of three increase in scatter [Townsend et al., 1989]. The success of this work at Hammersmith Hospital led to the design and appearance of the first commercial multi-ring scanner with retractable septa, the ECAT 953B from Siemens/CTI PET Systems (CPS), in 1990. The ECAT 953B opened up the possibility, for the first time, of performing PET studies in either 2D or 3D on the same scanner. Since 1991, with the exception of the ECAT ART and EXACT3D, all commercial, multi-ring scanners have been equipped with retractable septa. The ECAT 953B was followed by the whole-body ECAT 951R, also with a 10 cm axial FOV, and subsequently by the EXACT [Wienhard et al., 1992], the EXACT HR [Wienhard et al., 1994], and in 1995 the EXACT HR+ [Brix et al., 1997], all from CPS, with 15 cm FOVs. In 1992, General Electric Medical Systems announced the ADVANCE whole-body PET scanner with a 15 cm FOV [DeGrado et al., 1994], and in 1993 they marketed the NaI(Tl)-based QUEST scanner developed by UGM Medical Systems, the first commercial fully 3D PET scanner without septa, now available with a 25 cm axial FOV. The QUEST is based on pioneering work done with the PENN-PET system [Karp et al., 1990]. In 1994, following original work on a rotating partial ring tomograph [Townsend et al., 1993], CPS announced the first commercial fully 3D rotating scanner, the ECAT ART, which acquires and reconstructs PET data in 3D [Bailey et al., 1997]. More recently, a new design of septaless, multi-ring scanner, the EXACT3D, with 48 detector rings covering a 24 cm axial FOV, has been installed at Hammersmith Hospital in London [Jones et al., 1996].

Many of the early studies comparing 2D and 3D PET were carried out on the ECAT 953B [Townsend et al., 1991], although other centers also started to explore the potential of 3D PET [Cherry et al., 1991]. Difficulties that were encountered in this early work, some of which still limit the wider application of 3D PET, include the complexity of the reconstruction algorithm, the long reconstruction times, the large size data sets, the high levels of scatter, and validation of procedures for attenuation correction and 3D normalization. Although widely-used in brain mapping studies where only relative blood flow changes are required, 3D methodology has been applied only to a limited extent to neuroreceptor ligand studies [Trébossen et al., 1998] owing to a general concern over quantitative accuracy. Quantitation of 3D methodology in the thorax for absolute myocardial blood flow measurements, and in the thorax and abdomen for tumour uptake values in oncology applications still awaits further validation. Advances in the development of 3D PET methodology which will be discussed in detail in subsequent chapters of this monograph, have taken place in a number of these areas.

Reconstruction algorithms

Since 1992, the reprojection algorithm [Kinahan and Rogers, 1989] has emerged as the most widely-used 3D reconstruction algorithm and is based on an extension of standard 2D filtered backprojection to three dimensions. The algorithm uses the three-dimensional filter originally derived by Colsher [1980] within the context of a dual-head rotating gamma camera. The reprojection algorithm incorporates a preliminary step in which projections that are partially-measured because of the truncated cylindrical geometry of the multi-ring scanner are completed by forward projecting through an initial, low statistics image. This initial image is obtained from a reconstruction of the completely-measured, direct projections only. A version of the reprojection algorithm, or 3DRP, has been implemented on all commercially-available multi-ring PET scanners. As an alternative to the full 3D reconstruction algorithm, a 3D data set may be rebinned into a 2D data set by making certain approximations, and then reconstructed using a 2D reconstruction algorithm. Until recently, the most widely-used rebinning algorithm was single-slice rebinning (SSRB) [Daube-Witherspoon and Muehllehner, 1987], which assigned an oblique line of response to the mid transaxial slice, thereby introducing axial and transaxial blurring artifacts into the reconstructed image. There has been increased interest in using rebinning algorithms with the development of Fourier rebinning, FORE [Defrise, 1995]. Although still an approximation, FORE offers a more accurate approach to the rebinning procedure.

Reconstruction times

In establishing 3D PET as a practical alternative to standard 2D, a major difficulty has been the time required to reconstruct a single frame of data. As originally implemented on a SUN SparcStation 1, the 3D reprojection algorithm took six hours to reconstruct a 128x128x31 image from 7.8 million LORs. A comparable reconstruction in 2D took two minutes for 0.5 million LORs. However, the rapid progress in hardware in the past five years has resulted in reconstruction times under ten minutes per time frame. This dramatic improvement has been achieved by parallelizing the algorithm to run on multiple processors, generally i860-based systems. Nevertheless, as the reconstruction time has decreased, the data set size has increased due to an increase in both the number of detector rings and the number of crystals per ring. The 32-ring EXACT HR+ can, for example, acquire over 150 Mbytes for a single frame (85 million LORs). A reconstruction time for the 3D reprojection algorithm of 9 minutes is achieved with an array of eight i860 processors, after angular averaging and radial trimming has been applied to reduce the sinogram size. Similar times are reported for the 18-ring ADVANCE scanner which uses nine i860 processors to give a reconstruction time of 8 minutes. Generally, data sets acquired in 3D are 8-12 times larger than 2D data sets and they require 6-8 times longer than 2D to reconstruct.

Scatter correction

A number of different scatter correction techniques have been developed in the past few years, and results have been published in particular for the convolution-subtraction method [Bailey and Meikle, 1994], the dual energy window approach [Grootoonk et al., 1992; Bendriem et al., 1993], and more recently for the model-based method [Ollinger, 1994; Watson et al., 1996]. Results have been published [Townsend et al., 1994] from studies with the Utah phantom (described in Chapter 3) comparing convolution-subtraction and dual energy window scatter correction techniques which indicate that, in most studies to date, the background in 3D after scatter correction is reduced below that generally accepted in 2D (without correction). A major concern with the more open geometry of 3D systems is the influence of scatter and randoms from activity outside the FOV. Results from a study which simulates the effect of high levels of activity just outside the FOV, such as that measuring cerebral oxygen utilization by inhalation of radioactive gas suggest that the dual-energy window approach is effective in correcting for the scatter arising from activity outside the FOV.

Normalization

Considerable effort has been devoted to developing a satisfactory procedure for 3D normalization. Correction factors are required for effects due to the ring geometry of the scanner, the varying sensitivities of the different crystals, and interference effects dependent upon the position of the crystals within a block. Various investigators have proposed different source distributions with which to measure these effects, including a uniform cylinder, rotating rod sources, a rotating plane source, and a travelling line source. The difficulty is to design a source which is representative of actual source distributions (i.e. the brain or the heart), but which introduces minimal scatter. Significant scatter, such as that which arises with a uniform cylinder in 3D, can affect the estimate of crystal efficiencies. A completely satisfactory procedure for 3D normalization has yet to be developed.

Attenuation correction

Attenuation correction is an essential step in PET quantitation since typically more than 60% of all emitted photons interact with tissue. The correction requires a map of linear attenuation coefficients (μ-map) at 511 keV which can be either measured with an external source, or calculated from a knowledge of the boundaries of the attenuating medium. The challenge is to compromise between the accuracy of the correction, the noise propagation introduced by this process, and the possibility of mismatch between the true μ-map and the measured or calculated μ-map. While relatively straightforward for brain imaging, the measurement of accurate, low noise attenuation correction factors is somewhat more problematic for heart imaging. Whole-body imaging presents even greater difficulties because of the limited time available to acquire transmission data at each bed position. The standard technique for measuring attenuation correction factors is to acquire a transmission scan in 2D using rotating ^{68}Ge rod sources. The reconstructed transmission images are stacked to form a 3D volume, from which the full set of 3D attenuation correction factors can be obtained by reprojection. The advantage of acquiring the transmission scan with septa extended is that higher activity rod sources can be used without causing excessive deadtime problems in the detectors close to the sources. Scanners without septa, such as the ECAT ART, QUEST and the EXACT3D cannot acquire transmission scans in 2D and thus either lower activity rod sources or point sources [deKemp and Nahmias, 1994] must be used. The advantage of point sources is that they do not have to be positron-emitting isotopes to permit source localization. In addition, high count rates can be achieved with proper collimation of the source and shielding of the detector close to the source, and the recent use of 662 keV gammas from ^{137}Cs point sources for PET transmission scanning has dramatically improved the quality of transmission images. ^{137}Cs sources for attenuation correction measurements are now standard on the QUEST and the EXACT3D and under development for the ART. The measurements with ^{137}Cs sources must be scaled from 662 keV to 511 keV, and scatter correction remains an issue with singles scanning.

Summary

In the past ten or so years, 3D PET methodology has been the focus of a considerable amount of effort. Even though the first "3D ready" multi-ring scanners appeared as early as 1990, software which addressed the issues discussed above was not available for commercial multi-ring scanners until around 1993. Even today, hardware and software techniques for 3D PET are still evolving, and the aim of this monograph is to review the basic methodology and current status. In subsequent chapters, the mathematical basis of 3D reconstruction will be described in detail (Chapter 2), and the different procedures by which quantitative PET imaging is performed in 3D will be discussed in Chapter 3. Current scanner designs and the performance that can be achieved compared with standard 2D PET is the topic of Chapter 4, and in Chapter 5, the areas in which 3D PET methodology is being actively applied will be reviewed. The monograph concludes with a brief look into the future prospects of 3D PET imaging.

References

Allemand R, Gresset C, Vacher J. Potential advantages of a cesium fluoride scintillator for a time of flight positron camera. J Nucl Med 1980;21:153-155.

Bailey DL and Meikle SR. A convolution-subtraction scatter correction method for 3D PET. Phys Med Biol 1994;39:412-424.

Bailey DL, Young H, Bloomfield PM, Meikle SR, Glass D, Myers MJ, Spinks TJ, Watson CC, Luk P, Peters M, Jones T. ECAT ART - a continuosly rotating PET camera:

performance characteristics, inital clinical studies, and installation considerations in a nuclear medicine department. Eur J Nucl Med 1997;24(1):5-15.

Bendriem B, Trebossen R, Froulin V, Syrota A. A PET scatter correction using simultaneous acquisitions with low and high lower energy thresholds. IEEE Medical Imaging Conference Record 1993;3:1779-1783.

Brix G, Zaers J, Adam L-E, Bellemann ME, Ostertag H, Trojan H, Haberkorm U, Doll J, Oberdorfer F, Lorenz WJ. Performance evaluation of a whole-body PET scanner using the NEMA protocol. J Nucl Med 1997;38(10):1614-1623.

Casey ME and Nutt R. A multicrystal two-dimensional BGO detector system for positron emission tomography. IEEE Trans Nucl Sci 1986;NS-33:460-463.

Cherry SR, Dahlbom M, Hoffman EJ. Three-dimensional positron emission tomography using a conventional multislice tomograph without septa. J Comput Assist Tomogr 1991;15:655-668.

Cho ZH, Faruhki MR. Bismuth germanate as a potential scintillation detector in positron cameras. J Nucl Med 1977;18:840-844.

Colsher JG. Fully three-dimensional positron emission tomography. Phys Med Biol 1980;20:103-115.

Dahlbom M, Mandelkern MA, Hoffman EJ, Ricci AR, Barton JB. Hybrid Mercuric iodide HgI_2 - gadolinium orthosilicate (GSO) detector for PET. IEEE Trans Nucl Sci 1985;32:533-537.

Daube-Witherspoon ME and Muehllehner G. Treatment of axial data in three-dimensional PET. J Nucl Med 1987;28:1717-1724.

DeGrado TR, Turkington TG, Williams JJ, Stearns CW, Hoffman JM, Coleman RE. Performance characteristics of a whole-body PET scanner. J Nucl Med 1994;35:1398-1406.

deKemp RA, Nahmias C. Attenuation correction in PET using single photon transmission measurement. Med Phys 1994;21:771-778.

Defrise M. A factorization method for the 3D x-ray transform. Inverse Problems 11 1995;983-994.

Grootoonk S, Spinks TJ, Jones T, Michel C, Bol A. Correction for scatter using a dual energy window technique with a tomograph operating without septa. IEEE Medical Imaging Conference Record 1992;2:1569-1573.

Jones T, Bailey DL, Bloomfield PM, Spinks TJ, Jones W, Vaigneur K, Reed J, Young J, Newport D, Moyers C, Casey ME, Nutt R. Performance characteristics and novel design aspects of the most sensitive PET camera built for high temporal and spatial resolution. J Nucl Med 1996;37(5):85P.

Karp J, Muehllehner G, Mankoff DA, Ordonez CE, Ollinger JM, Daube-Witherspoon ME, Haigh AT, Beerbohm DJ. Continuous-slice PENN-PET: a positron tomograph with volume imaging capability. J Nucl Med 1990;31:617-627.

Kinahan PE and Rogers JG. Analytic three-dimensional image reconstruction using all detected events. IEEE Trans Nucl Sci 1989;NS-36:964-968.

Laval M, Moszynski M, Allemand R, Cormoreche E, Guinet P, Odru R, Vacher J. Barium fluoride - Inorganic scintillator for subnanosecond timing. Nucl Inst Meth 1983;206:169-176.

Mazoyer B, Trebossen R, Schoukroun C, Verrey B, Syrota A, Vacher J, Lemasson P, Monnet O, Bouvier A, Lecomte JL. Physical characteristics of TTV03, a new high spatial resolution time-of-flight positron tomograph. IEEE Trans Nucl Sci 1990;37:778-782.

Muehllehner G. Positron camera with extended counting rate capability. J Nucl Med 1975;16:653-657.

Ollinger JM. Evaluation of a model-based scatter correction for fully 3D PET. IEEE Medical Imaging Conference Record 1994;2:1264-1268.

Trebossen R, Bendriem B, Ribeiro MJ, Fontaine A, Frouin V, Remy P. Validation of the 3D acquisition mode in PET for the quantitation of the F-18 fluoradopa uptake in the striatum. J Cereb Blood Flow Metab 1998: in press.

Townsend DW, Frey P, Jeavons AP, Reich G, Tochon-Danguy HJ, Donath A, Christin A, Schaller G. High density avalanche chamber (HIDAC) positron camera. J Nucl Med 1987;28:1554-1562.

Townsend DW, Spinks TJ, Jones T, Geissbuhler A, Defrise M, Gilardi MC, Heather J. Three-dimensional reconstruction of PET data from a multi-ring camera. IEEE Trans Nucl Sci 1989;36:1056-1065.

Townsend DW, Geissbuhler A, Defrise M, Hoffman EJ, Spinks TJ, Bailey DL, Gilardi MC, Jones T. Fully three-dimensional reconstruction for a PET camera with retractable septa. IEEE Trans Med Imaging 1991;10(4):505-512.

Townsend DW, Wensween M, Byars LG, Geissbuhler A, Tochon-Danguy HJ, Christin A, Defrise M, Bailey DL, Grootoonk S, Donath A, Nutt R. A rotating PET scanner using BGO block detectors: design, performance and applications. J Nucl Med 1993;34(8):1367-1376.

Townsend DW, Choi Y, Sashin D, Mintun MA, Grootoonk S, Bailey DL. An investigation of practical scatter correction techniques for 3D PET. J Nucl Med Supplement 1994;35(5):50P.

Watson CC, Newport D, Casey ME. A single scatter simulation technique for scatter correction in three-dimensional PET. In: Grangeat P, Amans JL, editors. Three-dimensional image reconstruction in radiology and nuclear medicine. Dordrecht, The Netherlands: Kluwer, 1996:255-268.

Wienhard K, Eriksson L, Grootoonk S, Casey M, Pietrzyk U, Heiss W-D. Performance evaluation of the positron scanner ECAT EXACT. J Comput Assist Tomogr 1992;16(5):804-813.

Wienhard K, Dahlbom M, Eriksson L, Michel C, Bruckbauer T, Pietrzyk U, Heiss WD. The ECAT EXACT HR: performance of a new high resolution positron scanner. J Comput Assist Tomogr 1994;18:110-118.

Chapter 2. DATA ACQUISITION AND IMAGE RECONSTRUCTION FOR 3D PET

Michel Defrise[1] and Paul Kinahan[2]

[1]Division of Nuclear Medicine, Free University of Brussels (VUB), Belgium
[2]PET Facility, Department of Radiology, University of Pittsburgh, USA

The purpose of this chapter is to explain the underlying concepts of the most common image reconstruction methods. The question to be answered in this chapter is: how can we use the additional information from a 3D PET scan (as compared to a 2D scan) to improve the signal to noise ratio in the reconstructed image?

The first section describes the acquisition formats unique to 3D PET imaging. With this background, we next review well-known image reconstruction methods used in 2D PET imaging. We will then show in the third section how these 2D methods are extended to the more complex case of 3D image reconstruction. Some alternative 3D reconstruction methods are described in the fourth section. Finally, the last section briefly discusses the effect of the 3D data acquisition and image reconstruction on image variance.

3D PET Data Acquisition

THE LINE-INTEGRAL APPROXIMATION

For the block-type of PET scanner, a line-of-response (LOR) is usually regarded as the 'tube' that connects two individual scintillator crystals, as illustrated in fig. 2.1. In the absence of effects such as attenuation and scatter, the number of coincident events detected in a fixed time is proportional to the integral of the tracer concentration along the LOR. In an idealized (noiseless) case we can write this as,

$$\sum_{\mathrm{LOR}} (\mathrm{events}) \propto \int_{\mathrm{LOR}} d\mathbf{x}\, f(\mathbf{x}) \qquad (2.1)$$

where the function $f(\mathbf{x})$ represents the 3D tracer distribution. In practice, equation 2.1 is only true on average due to the stochastic nature of positron emission and annihilation photon detection.

A more accurate model is to assume that the sum of events for an LOR is a realization of a random distribution according to a probability distribution function (PDF). The PDF may be known or be assumed known, and the line-integral represents the mean or expected value, as given in equation 2.2.

B. Bendriem and D.W. Townsend (eds.) The Theory and Practice of 3D PET, 11-53.

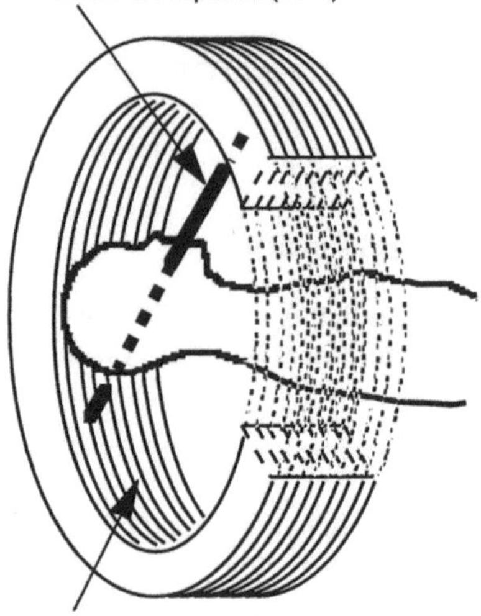

Figure 2.1 Schematic of a multi-ring PET scanner showing a single LOR intersecting the patient in the field of view corresponding to two detector elements.

$$E\left[\sum_{\text{LOR}}(\text{events})\right] = c\int_{\text{LOR}} d\mathbf{x}\, f(\mathbf{x})\,. \tag{2.2}$$

The PDF is usually assumed to be a Poisson distribution. This statistical approach will be discussed below.

DATA FORMATS

There are two different methods of accumulating event information during a PET scan. In the first, and more common, method a large array in computer memory is allocated such that there is an array element for each LOR that will be measured during the PET scan. Initially all of the array elements are set to 0. For each coincident event that is detected during the scan, the array element corresponding to the LOR is incremented by 1. This type of an array, which stores the total counts as a function of some variable such as position or energy, is called a *histogram*, and the individual storage elements are called *bins*. In PET imaging, the value of each bin represents the total sum of events along the corresponding LOR.

In the second method, event information is stored in a list-type format on an event-by-event basis as the events are detected. In *list mode* acquisition each entry contains information about an individual coincident event. List mode data are then typically reprocessed, or *rebinned*, by sorting the events into a histogram after the data acquisition is completed.

In many 2D PET imaging protocols the histogram format can be a much more compact form of data representation than list-mode format, as the average numbers of events per LOR is often greater than 1. In some 3D imaging protocols, however, the number of LORs, and thus the size of the histograms, is an order of magnitude larger than in 2D, leading to histograms that have an average number of events per LOR much less than 1. In these cases the list-mode format is usually more compact for data acquisition, although the event data must eventually be rebinned into histograms prior to reconstruction by the algorithms described later in this chapter. It should be noted that histogramming typically involves some loss of information, as the histogram bins only represent the total *number* of events that have been grouped together based upon common characteristics. For PET imaging, the common characteristics are typically chosen to be the pair of detectors in coincidence (the LOR index) *if* the deposited energy is within a pre-specified range. Other information, such as the energy and the order of occurrence, are lost during the binning process.

From this point we assume the data are in histogram format as a necessary first step for the image reconstruction algorithms. A useful idealized format for the histogrammed data is to assume the histogram bin values correspond to line integrals through the original object. The collection of all line-integrals parallel to a given direction is called a *projection*.

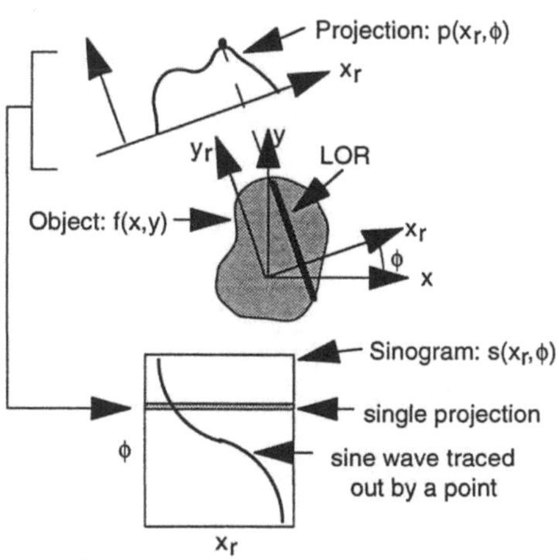

Figure 2.2 Idealized description of a one-dimensional projection of a 2D object as the collection of all parallel line-integrals for an angle ϕ relative to the scanner. The relation of a projection to the sinogram is also shown.

In 2D imaging the data representation can be parameterized in different manners, here we use the rotated coordinates illustrated in fig. 2.2, and the projection data, $p(x_r, \phi)$, are described by the integral,

$$p(x_r, \phi) = \int_{-\infty}^{\infty} dy_r \, f(x, y), \tag{2.3}$$

where (x_r, y_r) are rotated from (x, y) by an azimuthal angle ϕ relative to the scanner,

$$\begin{bmatrix} x \\ y \end{bmatrix} = \begin{bmatrix} \cos\phi & -\sin\phi \\ \sin\phi & \cos\phi \end{bmatrix} \begin{bmatrix} x_r \\ y_r \end{bmatrix}. \tag{2.4}$$

In the discrete form mandated in practice, we use the notation p_{ik} for the projection data with the transverse distance given by $x_r = i\,\Delta x_r$ and azimuthal angle given by $\phi = k\,\Delta\phi$, and *i*, *k*, are integer indices. This format can be easily expanded for use with 3D PET imaging as we will show below.

The 2D data, equation 2.3, can be stored and displayed as a 2D array indexed by x_r and ϕ. These arrays are called *sinograms* since a point source in the scanner's FOV traces out a sine wave pattern, as illustrated in fig. 2.2. The data are only stored for the range $0 \le \phi < \pi$, since for $\pi \le \phi < 2\pi$ the projections have a symmetry given by, $p(x_r, \phi + \pi) = p(-x_r, \phi)$. A sinogram can also be considered to be the 2D Radon transform of an object, which we will not discuss further but is well described by Deans [Deans, 1983].

In 3D PET imaging, projections are 2D sets of parallel line-integrals with a given azimuthal angle ϕ and co-polar angle θ, as illustrated in fig. 2.3. Note that in fig. 2.3 the scanner *z*-axis is vertical following the usual mathematical convention, whereas in fig. 2.1 it is shown in its true horizontal position.

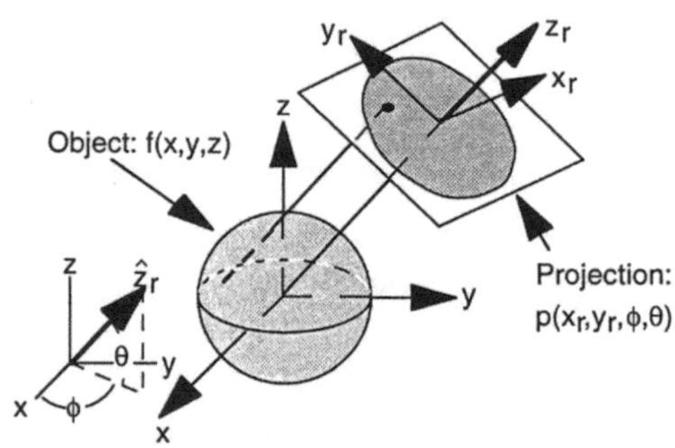

Figure 2.3 Definition of a 2D projection as the collection of all parallel line-integrals for azimuthal angle ϕ and co-polar angle θ relative to the scanner coordinates.

The equation describing the 2D projections is a straightforward generalization of equation 2.4 to

$$p(x_r, y_r, \phi, \theta) = \int_{-\infty}^{\infty} dz_r \, f(x, y, z) \tag{2.5}$$

where the 3D rotation of coordinates is given by,

$$\begin{bmatrix} x \\ y \\ z \end{bmatrix} = \begin{bmatrix} -\sin\phi & -\cos\phi\sin\theta & \cos\phi\cos\theta \\ \cos\phi & -\sin\phi\sin\theta & \sin\phi\cos\theta \\ 0 & \cos\theta & \sin\theta \end{bmatrix} \begin{bmatrix} x_r \\ y_r \\ z_r \end{bmatrix} \tag{2.6}$$

Note that when $\theta = 0$, equations 2.5 and 2.6 reduce to the 2D case given in equations 2.3 and 2.4 for the 2D plane given by $z = y_r$.

The projection data are now four dimensional in nature, and the discrete form of the projection data for individual LOR sums is given by p_{ijkl}, where i, j, k, and l are integer indices, and

$$\begin{aligned} x_r &= i\,\Delta x_r \\ y_r &= j\,\Delta y_r \\ \phi &= k\,\Delta\phi \\ \theta &= l\,\Delta\theta \end{aligned}$$

In contrast with 2D PET imaging, there are two formats used for storing the four dimensional projection data. These are illustrated in fig. 2.4 for a small spherical object which is located off-center to illustrate the relationship between the two formats. These modes are called by different names, here we label them as projection mode (fig. 2.4(a)) and oblique sinogram mode (fig. 2.4(b)).

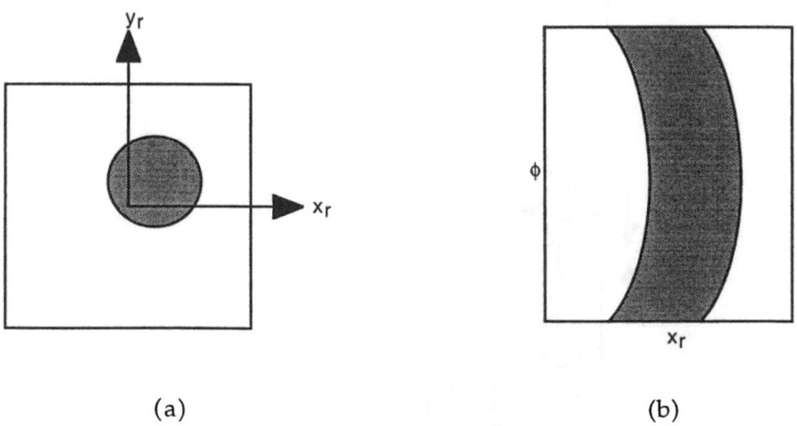

Figure 2.4 The two formats for storing the four dimensional projection data collected in 3D PET imaging. (a) projection format (also shown in fig. 2.3), shown for one value of (ϕ, θ). (b) Oblique sinogram format, shown for one value of (y_r, θ).

Both formats represent the same data, but with a different ordering of the parameters as can be seen by comparing figs. 2.4(a) and 2.4(b). The choice of which format to use is usually based on what is most convenient for a data processing or analysis procedure. The exact relationship between these two formats is described in the next section.

DATA SAMPLING AND REDUCTION

Data sampling. The most common type of 3D PET tomograph is the cylindrical multi-ring block-detector PET scanner. These scanners have intrinsic data sampling patterns determined by the geometrical arrangement of the scintillation detectors [Townsend and Defrise, 1993]. For volumetric sampling, we use the scanner model outlined in fig. 2.5.

In this model the active scanner forms a cylindrical surface subdivided into uniform detector elements of area $\Delta d_t \times \Delta d_z$ in the transverse and axial directions. In the transverse direction the sampling is a fan-beam pattern, with equal angles of $\Delta d_t / 2R_D$ between the fan rays, as shown in fig. 2.6(a).

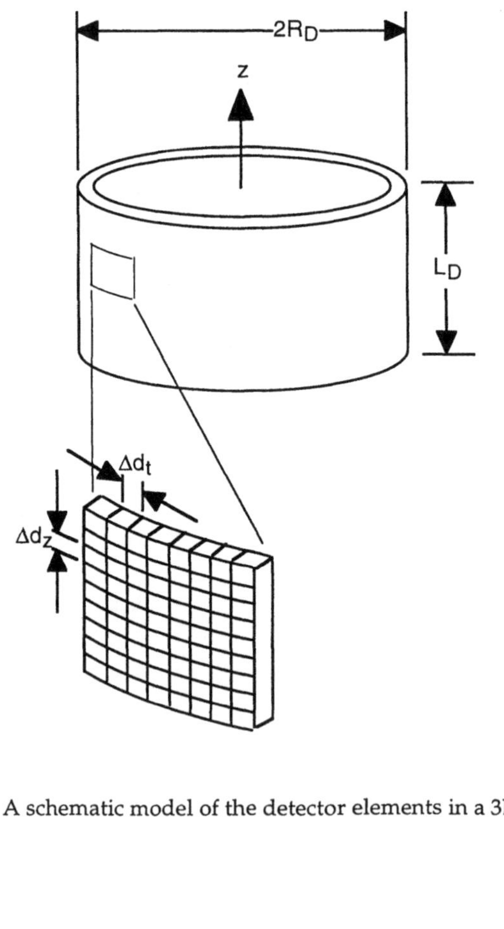

Figure 2.5 A schematic model of the detector elements in a 3D PET scanner.

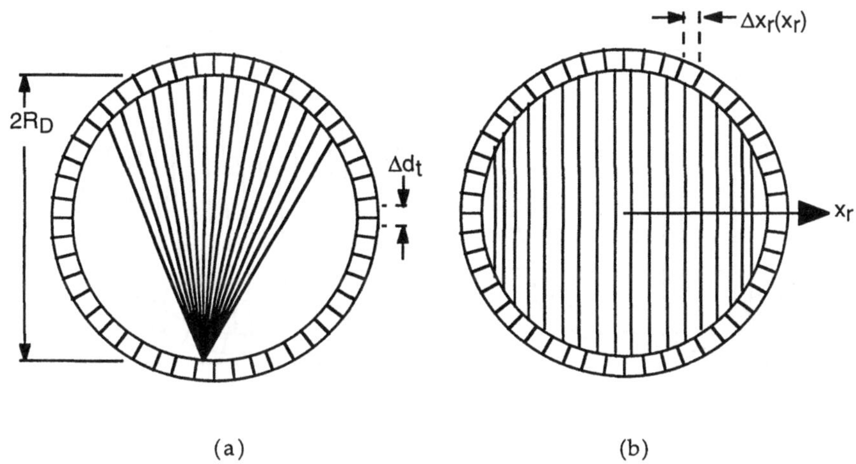

Figure 2.6 Cross-section of a cylindrical tomograph with detector radius R_D showing the transverse sampling patterns. (a) The intrinsic equiangular fan-beam pattern. (b) The approximately equi-spaced parallel-beam pattern often used in practice.

The usual practice, however, is to treat the data as a parallel-beam pattern as shown in fig. 2.6(b), which also shows that the actual ray-spacing is given by

$$\Delta x_r = \Delta d_t \sqrt{1-\left(\frac{x_r}{R_D}\right)^2}$$

where Δd_t is the center-to-center spacing of the detector elements in the transverse direction given by $\Delta d_t = 2\pi R_D / N_d$ and N_d is the number of detector elements within a single transaxial ring. This leads to decreasing ray-spacing with increasing transverse distance from the center. In cases where $|x_r| << R_D$, the approximation $\Delta x_r \approx \Delta d_t$ of uniform spacing is usually made, otherwise the data must be interpolated to uniform spacing along the x_r direction. This correction is referred to as the *arc correction*.

To understand the sampling pattern in a sinogram, consider fig. 2.7, which shows the correspondence between sets of parallel LORs and the LOR locations on a sinogram for a scanner with an even number of transverse detector elements N_d. In this manner, the number of angular samples, N_ϕ, in the range $0 \le \phi < \pi$, is equal to the number of detectors N_d. As can be seen from fig. 2.7, the x_r coordinate of the bin centers for adjacent rows is offset by $\Delta x_r/2$, and the number of transverse samples N_{xr}, is at most $N_d/2$, but is typically limited to approximately one-half of that, depending on the ratio of the scanner and FOV diameters. If adjacent rows of the sinogram are interleaved, the transverse sampling rate is doubled and the angular sampling rate is halved. The effect of this interleaving is a slight alternating error of $\pm\Delta\phi/4$ in the assumed ϕ coordinate of the bin center. With this sampling pattern there are $N_\phi = N_d/2$ angular and $N_{xr} \approx N_d/2$ transverse samples, with an angular bin size of $\Delta\phi = \pi/N_\phi$ and a transverse bin size of $\Delta x_r = 2R/N_{xr} \approx \Delta d_t/2$.

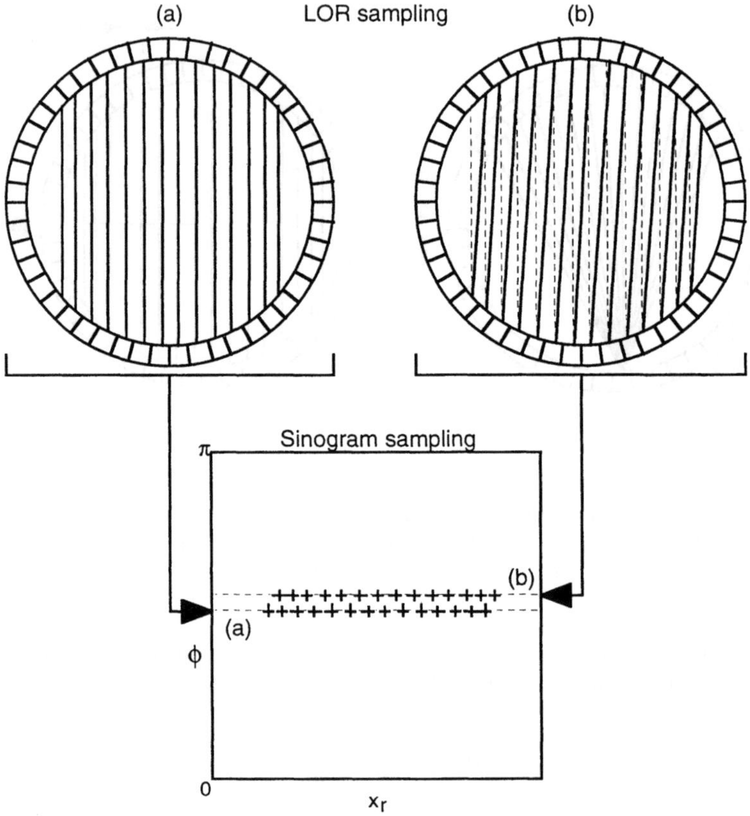

Figure 2.7 sinogram sampling pattern for a scanner with an even number of detector elements. In (b) the LORs are moved by shifting only one of the two detector endpoints, and the previous LORs are indicated by dashed lines. Thus, for (b) an LOR samples the exact center of the FOV, while for (a) the two central LORs straddle the center of the FOV. This leads to an offset in the transverse sampling pattern for adjacent rows.

In the axial direction, the intrinsic sampling is determined by the center-to-center spacing Δd_z of the detector elements in the axial direction, where $\Delta d_z = L_D / N_R$. For a scanner with N_R detector rings, there are N_R^2 possible ring combinations for oblique LORs, as shown in fig. 2.8. These combinations can be indexed by (ring1, ring2) $((r_1, r_2))$ coordinates or by $(z, \Delta r)$ coordinates, with an average axial coordinate $z = (r_1 + r_2)/2$ and ring difference $\Delta r = (r_1 - r_2)$.

In general, the (y_r, θ) coordinates for the projection format defined in fig. 2.3 do not correspond to true LORs. The relationship between projections and oblique sinograms is given by

$$p(x_r, y_r, \phi, \theta) = s(x_r, \phi, z, \Delta r)$$

where

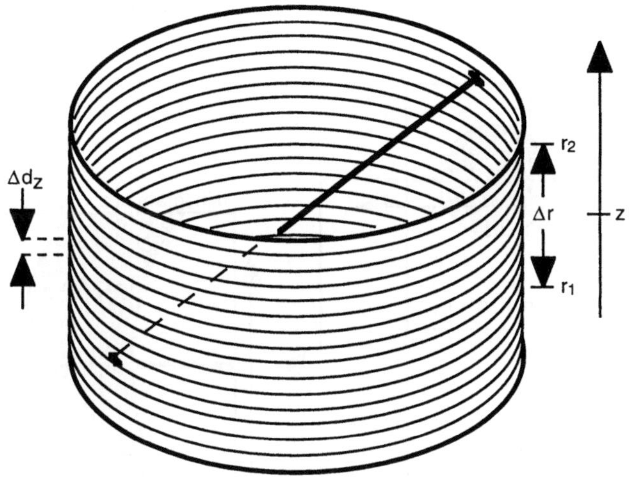

Figure 2.8 The $(z, \Delta r)$ coordinates of an oblique sinogram containing the indicated LOR for an N_R-ring PET scanner.

$$y_r = z\cos\theta$$

where,

$$\tan\theta = \frac{\Delta r}{2\sqrt{R_D^2 - x_r^2}}$$

and R_D is the radius of the detector ring. When the radius of the FOV, R, and the maximum axial extent of the tomograph are small compared with R_D, $\tan\theta$ may be approximated with,

$$\tan\theta \approx \frac{\Delta r}{2R_D}$$

With this approximation, θ no longer depends upon the transverse coordinate x_r, and each row in the sinogram is a one-dimensional parallel projection. Thus, an oblique sinogram for a given $(z, \Delta r)$ can be formed by extracting a row of x_r values corresponding to $y_r = z\cos\theta$ (with $\theta \approx \arctan(\Delta r / 2R_D)$) and inserting the row at the ϕ coordinate of the original projection plane. This is illustrated in fig. 2.9.

If the approximations used above are not valid, the PET oblique sinogram data will require interpolation in order to obtain true parallel projections. From this point on we will assume that the 2D and 3D projections accurately reflect the true locations of the LORs.

Data reduction. The total size of a projection data set is given by $N_T \approx N_R{}^2 \times (N_d/2)^2 \times N_b$, where N_b is the number of bytes of storage per bin. With typical values of $N_R = 24$, $N_d = 512$, and $N_b = 2$, a single projection data set could potentially occupy approximately 50 to 100 Mbytes.

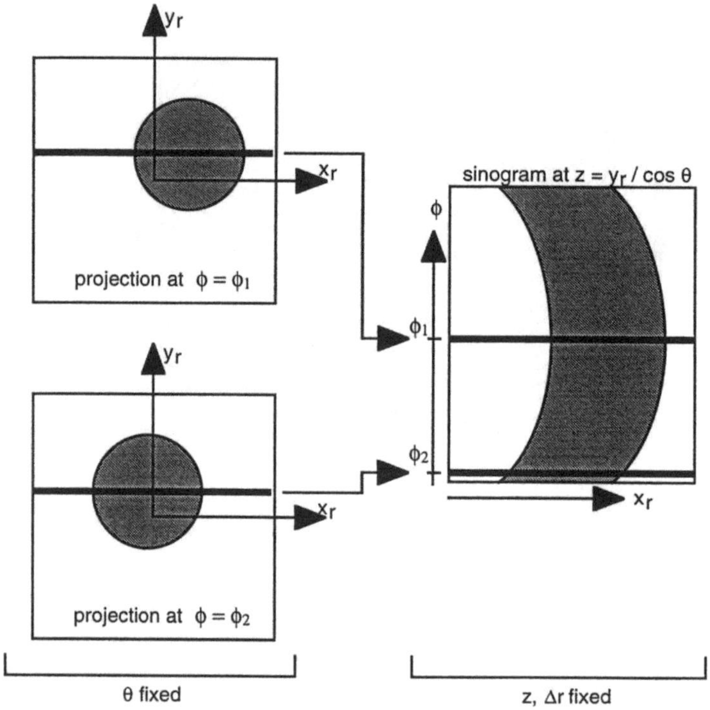

Figure 2.9 The correspondence between projections and oblique sinograms in the case where the approximations of $|x_r|, |\Delta r| << R_D$ are valid.

Due to the large size of a full 3D PET data set, the effects of reducing the data set size are important. To determine the smallest, but sufficient, data set size allowed by Shannon's sampling theorem, we start with the 2D PET imaging case with an intrinsic transverse sampling of Δx_r as described above. The maximum recoverable spatial frequency is then given by the Nyquist frequency of $\upsilon_N = 1/2\Delta x_r$. In the azimuthal direction, the samples are spaced farthest apart at the edge of the FOV, where we would like to constrain $\Delta\phi R \approx \Delta x_r$. In this case $\Delta x_r = 2R/N_{xr} \approx \Delta\phi R = (\pi / N_\phi R)$ and we have a consistency condition of $N_\phi \approx (\pi/2) N_{xr}$ [Natterer, 1986]. As discussed above the sampling pattern adopted in practice leads to $N_{xr} \approx N_\phi = N_d/2$ which is in good agreement with the consistency condition.

In practice, the maximum spatial frequency to be recovered is typically limited to some cut-off frequency $\upsilon_c < \upsilon_N$ to reduce the effect of statistical noise, as discussed in more detail below. In this case the number of angular samples can be reduced without significant loss in image resolution. The reduced number of angular samples N'_ϕ, is typically given by $N'_\phi = N_\phi \cdot 2^{-m}$, with $\Delta\phi' = \Delta\phi \cdot 2^m$, where $m = 0,1,2,\ldots$ is often called the *mashing* factor. For $m = 2$, for example, the data set size is reduced by a factor of 4. It is also possible to reduce the number of transverse samples N_{xr}, by increasing Δx_r, but image quality is more sensitive to this type of data reduction, and it is rarely done.

For 3D PET imaging the analysis to determine sufficient sampling in all 4 coordinates is more complex due to redundant sampling, as described below, and a full analysis has not been published. The number of samples in the (x_r, y_r) coordinates are generally not reduced from the intrinsic data sampling size. For the ϕ coordinate, mashing can be performed as described above. In the θ direction, however, the situation is somewhat more complex as there are additional free parameters. A useful conceptual tool is the 'Michelogram'[1] that graphically illustrates mashing in the θ coordinate, and is illustrated in fig. 2.10.

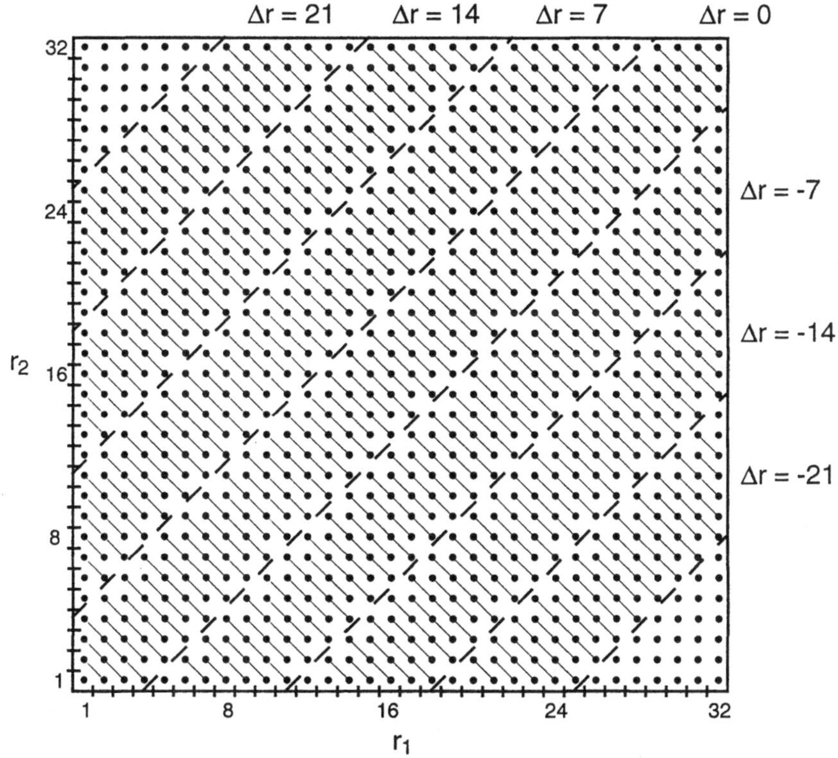

Figure 2.10 Illustration of the Michelogram for a hypothetical 32 ring scanner. Each dot represents the sinogram for the pair of rings (r_1, r_2). Sinograms with the same z value and adjacent θ values are grouped together to form wider bins in the θ direction. This grouping is shown by the diagonal lines connecting the dots. In this example, a span of 7 was chosen, resulting in 7 segments ($\Delta r = \{0, \pm 7, \pm 14, \pm 21\}$) and a $\Delta r_{\max}$ of 24.

---

[1]This notation was devised by Christian Michel of the Catholic University of Louvain, Belgium.

To reduce the number of θ samples, LORs adjacent in the θ direction are grouped together. The size, $\Delta\theta$, of the projection bin in the θ direction is called the 'span'. As fig. 2.10 also illustrates, the maximum value of Δr can also be reduced to a value less than $N_R - 1$, although there is a trade-off between overall sensitivity and reconstruction time. After choosing a maximum value of Δr, only certain spans are possible as the resulting N_θ must be integer-valued.

As a final point, we note that increasing $\Delta\theta$ may not necessarily lead to aliasing artifacts from under-sampling, as the image can be accurately reconstructed from just the direct projections (those with $\theta = 0$) using the 2D reconstruction methods described next. As $\Delta\theta$ is increased, however, the image will suffer from geometric distortions similar to those caused by the single-slice rebinning (SSRB) method described below.

Review of 2D image reconstruction

In this section we review well-known methods for inverting equation 2.1 for 2D PET imaging. There are several different ways to derive the equations used for 2D image reconstruction [Barrett and Swindell, 1981; Deans, 1983; Natterer, 1986]. We have chosen as a review of the 2D theory a derivation based on the central-section theorem that gives the most intuitive explanation. This approach is then extended to outline the key theoretical foundations of 3D image reconstruction.

THE 2D CENTRAL-SECTION THEOREM

For 2D PET imaging, we recall that the projection data are described by (repeating equations 2.3 and 2.4),

$$p(x_r,\phi) = \int_{-\infty}^{\infty} dy_r\, f(x,y) \tag{2.7}$$

where (x_r, y_r) is the rotated coordinate system given by,

$$\begin{bmatrix} x \\ y \end{bmatrix} = \begin{bmatrix} \cos\phi & -\sin\phi \\ \sin\phi & \cos\phi \end{bmatrix} \begin{bmatrix} x_r \\ y_r \end{bmatrix} \tag{2.8}$$

An important aspect of 2D PET imaging is that it can be approximated by a linear shift-invariant process. Shift-invariance is a property that will be more fully described below, but for now we note that an important consequence of shift-invariance is that the 1D Fourier transform of the projection data can be calculated. That is, we can compute,

$$P(\upsilon_{xr},\phi) = \int_{-\infty}^{\infty} dx_r\, e^{-2\pi i x_r \upsilon_{xr}}\, p(x_r,\phi) = F_1\{p(x_r,\phi)\} \tag{2.9}$$

where $F_1\{\cdot\}$ is defined as the 1D Fourier transform with respect to the first variable. We can achieve a key insight into the relation between the parallel projections and the tracer distribution *f(x,y)* by expanding the right hand side of equation 2.9,

$$
\begin{aligned}
P(\upsilon_{xr},\phi) &= \int_{-\infty}^{\infty} dx_r\, e^{-2\pi i x_r \upsilon_{xr}}\, p(x_r,\phi) \\
&= \int_{-\infty}^{\infty}\int_{-\infty}^{\infty} dx_r\, dy_r\, e^{-2\pi i x_r \upsilon_{xr}}\, f(x,y) \\
&= \int_{-\infty}^{\infty}\int_{-\infty}^{\infty} dx\, dy\, e^{-2\pi i \upsilon_{xr}(x\cos\phi + y\sin\phi)}\, f(x,y) \\
&= F(\upsilon_{xr}\cos\phi,\ \upsilon_{xr}\sin\phi)
\end{aligned}
\tag{2.10}
$$

where $F(\upsilon_x,\upsilon_y) = \int_{-\infty}^{\infty}\int_{-\infty}^{\infty} dx\, dy\, e^{-2\pi i(\upsilon_x x + \upsilon_y y)} f(x,y) = F_2\{f(x,y)\}$,

and $F_2\{\cdot\}$ is the 2D Fourier transform with respect to the first two variables.

The result of equation 2.10 shows that the 1D Fourier transform of a projection at an angle ϕ is equivalent to the value along a line through the origin (at the same angle) of the 2D Fourier transform of *f(x,y)*. More concisely,

$$
P(\upsilon_{xr},\phi) = F(\upsilon_x,\upsilon_y)\big|_{\upsilon_{yr}=0} \tag{2.11}
$$

This important result is known as the central-section theorem or the projection-slice theorem [Kak and Slaney, 1988], since the equivalence is for lines passing through the center of the 2D Fourier transform of *f(x,y)*, as illustrated in fig. 2.11.

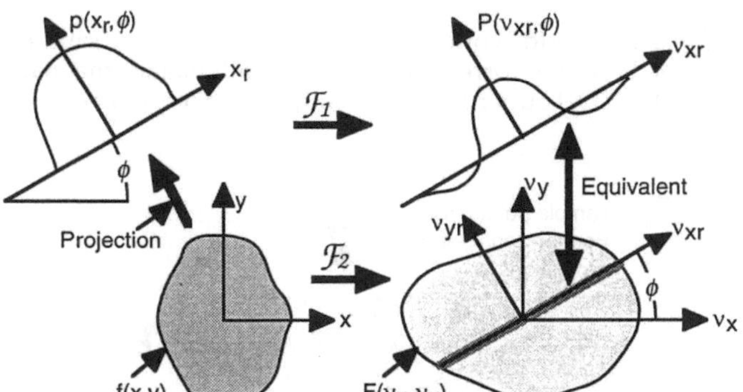

Figure 2.11 Illustration of the 2D central-section theorem.

The 2D central-section theorem establishes the following condition for necessary and sufficient data: In order to determine *f(x,y)*, we need $p(x_r,\phi)$ for all $|x_r| \le R$ and all $\phi: 0 \le \phi < \pi$. This follows since there is a one-to-one mapping from $F(\upsilon_x,\upsilon_y)$ to *f(x,y)*, and if $P(\upsilon_{xr},\phi)$ is known for all ϕ, then by the central-section theorem it is possible to determine $F(\upsilon_x,\upsilon_y)$ for all (υ_x,υ_y).

One method of image reconstruction, then, is to calculate $P(\upsilon_{xr},\phi)$ for all $\phi: 0 \leq \phi < \pi$, and 'place' these values in a 2D array representing $F(\upsilon_x,\upsilon_y)$, and then calculate the inverse 2D Fourier transform to estimate $f(x,y)$. This idea is illustrated in fig. 2.12.

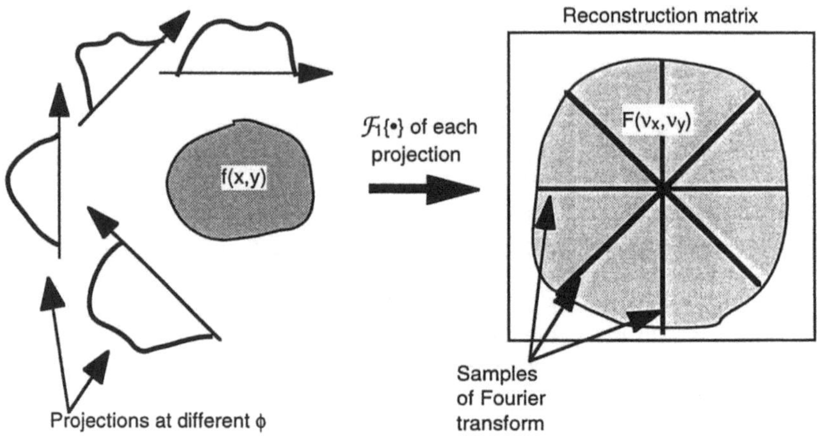

Figure 2.12 A method of 2D image reconstruction based on the central-section theorem. This method leads to over-sampling of the Fourier transform at the origin as described in the text.

The method of fig. 2.12 would work, except that we have over sampling at the origin, which somehow needs to be corrected for. To understand the nature of the over sampling, consider the 2D Fourier transform built up from discrete sample points as shown in fig. 2.13.

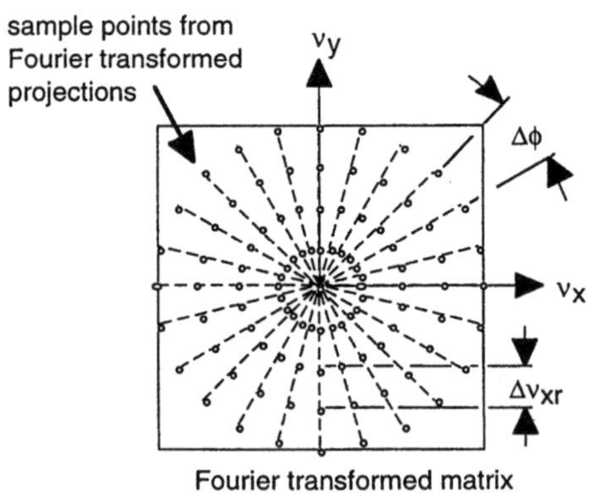

Figure 2.13 2D Fourier transform built up from discrete sample points from $P(\upsilon_{xr},\phi)$, the Fourier transform of the 1D projection data.

In fig. 2.13, the location of the sample points are given by $P(\upsilon_{xr},\phi) = P(i\Delta\upsilon_{xr}, k\Delta\phi)$, and as $\Delta\upsilon_{xr} \to 0$ and $\Delta\phi \to 0$, the density of sample points becomes proportional to $1/\upsilon$, where $\upsilon = |\bar{\upsilon}| = \sqrt{\upsilon_x^2 + \upsilon_y^2}$ is the radial coordinate in frequency space, and is also the Jacobian of the coordinate transform from rectangular to polar coordinates, that is, $d\upsilon_x\, d\upsilon_y = \upsilon\, d\upsilon\, d\phi$. This information about the sampling density will allow us to correctly normalize $F(\upsilon_x, \upsilon_y)$ and perform an inverse 2D Fourier transform to obtain $f(x,y)$.

2D IMAGE RECONSTRUCTION BY FILTERED-BACKPROJECTION

As a preliminary step towards developing a 2D image reconstruction algorithm, we will first describe the operation of *backprojection*. This will lead us to an efficient method of placing the Fourier transform of the projection data into the 2D reconstruction array as illustrated in fig. 2.13. The backprojection operator can be considered as the adjoint to the forward projection done during the data acquisition process by the PET scanner. Mathematically backprojection is described by,

$$b(x,y) = \int_0^{\pi} d\phi\, p(x_r,\phi) \tag{2.12}$$

Backprojection is the most time consuming operation in image reconstruction due to the number of interpolation and array indexing steps. To calculate $b(x,y)$ for each point in a reconstruction array, equation 2.12 would have to be repeated for each point.

An efficient manner of backprojection is illustrated in fig. 2.14(a), where for a given ϕ, values of $p(x_r,\phi)$ are 'back-propagated' for each value of x_r in turn. The backprojected values increment the appropriate locations in the reconstruction array by the value of $p(x_r,\phi)$. By a corollary of the central-section theorem, this process is equivalent to placing the Fourier transformed values $P(\upsilon_{xr},\phi)$ into an array representing $F(\upsilon_x, \upsilon_y)$, as shown in fig. 2.14(b). This operation is then repeated for each ϕ to build up the complete 2D function $b(x,y)$.

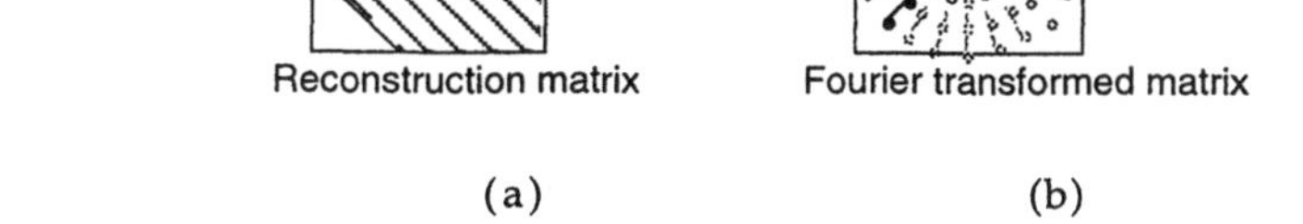

Figure 2.14 An efficient method of backprojection. (a) the back-propagation of the value $p(x_r,\phi)$ is done for each value of x_r for a fixed ϕ. (b) This backprojection for a single ϕ is equivalent to placing $P(\upsilon_{xr},\phi)$ into an array representing $F(\upsilon_x, \upsilon_y)$ at the same angle.

As an aside, we note that the backprojected image $b(x,y)$, can be considered the output of a linear shift-invariant imaging process. That is, if $h(x-x',y-y')$ is the 2D shift-invariant point-spread function (PSF) characterizing the response of the PET system at (x,y) to a point source at (x',y'), then,

$$b(x,y)=\int_{-\infty}^{\infty}\int_{-\infty}^{\infty}h(x-x',y-y')f(x',y')dx'\,dy'.$$

The PSF is called shift-invariant since the response at a point (x,y) to a point source at (x',y') depends only on the distances $(x-x')$, and $(y-y')$, so that,

$$b(x,y)=f(x,y)**h(x,y),$$

where '$**$' denotes the 2D convolution operator. As noted earlier, the property of shift-invariance also implies that we can easily calculate the Fourier transform of the projection data, a distinction that will become important in discussing the reconstruction of 3D PET data.

By comparing figs. 2.13 and 2.14 it is apparent that by computing the 2D Fourier transform of $b(x,y)$, we have the weighted version of the Fourier transform on the original function,

$$B(\upsilon_x,\upsilon_y)=F_2\{b(x,y)\}=F(\upsilon_x,\upsilon_y)\cdot(1/\upsilon) \tag{2.13}$$

An important insight is that the backprojection of data collected by a 2D PET scanner leads to the weighted sampling of the Fourier transform of the tracer distribution as described by equation 2.13. The goal of image reconstruction can thus be considered as properly normalizing the Fourier transform of the measured data so the correct inverse Fourier transform can be calculated. This is the approach we will take in describing 3D image reconstruction.

It is now possible to see that we can reconstruct $f(x,y)$ from the following equation,

$$f(x,y)=F_2^{-1}\left\{\upsilon F_2\left\{b(x,y)=\int_0^{\pi}d\phi\, p(x_r,\phi)\right\}\right\} \tag{2.14}$$

where $F_2^{-1}\{\cdot\}$ is the inverse 2D Fourier transform operator. This approach is known as the backprojection-filtering (BPF) method, where the projection data are first backprojected and then 'filtered' in frequency space by multiplication with the Jacobian υ $(0\le\upsilon<\infty)$, and finally the inverse 2D Fourier transform is calculated.

The most common 2D image reconstruction method is a variant of the BPF algorithm that takes advantage of the linearity of integral operators to interchange the ordering of filtering and backprojection, so that filtering of the one-dimensional projection is performed first to 'pre-correct' for the sampling of the 2D Fourier transform of the image. The second step is to then backproject the filtered projection, which results in an image where the blurring by the PSF has been properly corrected for. With this order of processing in mind, we can rewrite equation 2.14 as,

$$f(x,y) = \int_0^{\pi} \left[\int_{-\infty}^{\infty} d\upsilon_{xr}\, e^{2\pi i \upsilon_{xr} x_r} |\upsilon_{xr}| P(\upsilon_{xr},\phi) \right] d\phi \tag{2.15}$$

where the absolute value of $|\upsilon_{xr}|$ is used to allow integration from $-\infty$ to ∞. In this case the 1D filter term is a section through the center of the cone-shaped 2D υ filter $(0 \le \upsilon < \infty)$, and $|\upsilon_{xr}|$ is the well-known *ramp* filter. This reconstruction method is called, not surprisingly, the filtered-backprojection (FBP) algorithm, and consists of the following steps,

1 Fourier transform the projection $P(\upsilon_{xr},\phi) = F_1\{p(x_r,\phi)\}$ for a given ϕ

2 filter the projection in frequency space $P^F(\upsilon_{xr},\phi) = |\upsilon_{xr}| P(\upsilon_{xr},\phi)$

3 inverse Fourier transform the filtered projection $p^F(x_r,\phi) = F_1^{-1}\{P^F(\upsilon_{xr},\phi)\}$

4 backproject the filtered projection $f(x,y) = f(x,y) + \Delta\phi \cdot p^F(x_r,\phi)$ for all x_r

5 repeat steps 1-4 for each $\phi: 0 \le \phi < \pi$

The exact inversion of equation 2.13 is not possible in practice due to two factors. The first factor arises from the discrete sampling necessary in practice, which sets a maximum bound on the frequency information that can be recovered. According to Shannon's sampling theorem, the maximum recoverable frequency is the Nyquist frequency $\upsilon_N = 1/2\Delta x_r$. Trying to recover higher frequencies in the reconstruction will result in aliasing artifacts. The second limiting factor is the presence of statistical noise. The power spectrum of the exact, noise-free, projections typically decreases more rapidly than the corresponding power spectrum of the statistical noise. Thus, above a certain frequency, which depends on the signal-to-noise ratio (SNR), the Fourier transform of $P(\upsilon_{xr},\phi)$ is dominated by noise, and the application of the ramp filter to higher frequencies results in amplification of the noise power, degrading the SNR of the reconstructed image.

To avoid these problems, a frequency low pass, or apodizing, window, $W(\upsilon_{xr})$, is used to eliminate any contributions from frequencies above a predetermined cut-off frequency υ_c. The appropriate choice of υ_c is determined by both the sampling distance (Δx_r) and the photon statistics. The choice of the apodizing window function $W(\upsilon_{xr})$ and υ_c will determine the spatial resolution of the reconstructed image, as well as its noise characteristics.

A typical window function used in PET reconstruction is the generalized Hamming window,

$$W_H(\upsilon_{xr}) = \begin{cases} \alpha + (1-\alpha)\cos\left(\dfrac{\pi\upsilon_{xr}}{\upsilon_c}\right), & |\upsilon_{xr}| < \upsilon_c \\ 0 & |\upsilon_{xr}| \ge \upsilon_c \end{cases} \tag{2.16}$$

where α $(0.5 \le \alpha \le 1.0)$ controls the shape of the window and $\upsilon_c \le \upsilon_N$ controls the maximum frequency as shown in fig. 2.15 for the ramp filter modified by the window function.

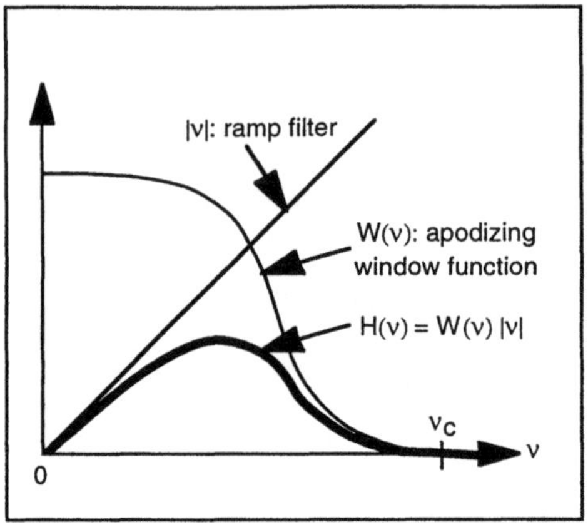

Figure 2.15 Modification of the ramp filter by multiplication with a Hamming window.

A considerable number of window functions have been evaluated in the literature, although the only significant properties are the frequency cut-off υ_c, and the shape of $W(\upsilon_{xr})$ as $\upsilon_{xr} \to \upsilon_c$.

With the use of the window function, the FBP algorithm becomes,

$$f(x,y) \approx \int_0^{\pi} d\phi\, F_1^{-1}\{W(\upsilon_{xr})|\upsilon_{xr}|F_1\{p(x_r,\phi)\}\} \tag{2.17}$$

where the equality has been replaced by an estimation due to the loss of high-frequency terms caused by the use of $W(\upsilon_{xr})$. Equation 2.17 summarizes the 2D FBP algorithm, which is the most common method of image reconstruction used in 2D PET imaging.

The final step is to form a volume image using 2D images. To do this, adjacent planes are imaged, usually with septa defining the adjacent planes. The planes are then each reconstructed separately, and then stacked together to form an image volume.

OTHER 2D RECONSTRUCTION METHODS

The FBP algorithm reviewed in the previous section is one of several well-known methods used in 2D image reconstruction. It is possible to divide 2D image reconstruction methods into two classes, transform and iterative. Transform methods are based on discrete implementations of analytic solutions similar to equation 2.12 and give a "one-step" solution, that is, the image estimate is directly calculated from the data. Iterative methods, on the other hand, incorporate the discrete nature of the data sampling and reconstruction problem and typically some statistical model of the data acquisition process. The systems of equations, however, are so large that these methods attempt to approach an acceptable solution by a series of successively refined estimations.

Transform Methods

All 2D transform methods can be related to the 2D FBP method, and one example we have already seen is the BPF method, where the backprojection and filtering steps are interchanged (equation 2.14). A commonly used variation is Convolution-backprojection (CBP), where filtering is done in projection space by convolution with the filter kernel. This is based on the Fourier-convolution theorem, which states that if:

$$h(x_r) = F_1^{-1}\{W(\upsilon_{xr})|\upsilon_{xr}|\}$$

then,

$$f(x,y) = \int_0^{\pi} d\phi \left[p(x_r,\phi) * h(x_r) \right]$$

where the $*$ operator denotes a one-dimensional convolution.

An alternative method is to directly place the Fourier transform of the projection data $P(\upsilon_{xr},\phi)$ into the reconstruction array by interpolation, and then compute the 2D inverse Fourier transform to estimate $f(x,y)$. In these 2D *Direct Fourier Methods,* interpolation is necessary for re-sampling from polar to rectangular grids (fig. 2.13). For Direct Fourier reconstruction methods, image quality is determined largely by the chosen trade-off between accuracy and computational speed, which depends on the interpolation algorithm used. Several interpolation algorithms have been implemented for image reconstruction [Cheung and Lewitt, 1991; Jackson et al., 1991], but a discussion of them is beyond the scope of this book.

Iterative methods:

In contrast to transform reconstruction methods, iterative methods attempt to progressively refine estimates of $f(x,y)$, rather than arriving at an estimate by direct inversion of the image transform. These methods allow a more accurate modeling of the data acquisition than the line-integral model of equation 2.1. In addition, the incorporation of an accurate model of the statistical noise can be a significant advantage. A further advantage of iterative methods is the ability to incorporate *a priori* information about the image into the reconstruction process. Such *a priori* information can be particularly useful in guiding the reconstruction algorithm towards an acceptable solution when the usual constraints provided by the data are weak, for example in the case of low SNR or poor sampling. One such constraint is non-negativity, which ensures that successive estimates of $f(x,y)$ are everywhere non-negative, which is reasonable since $f(x,y)$ represents tracer concentration. Another potential constraint is the inclusion of anatomical information obtained from X-ray CT or MRI studies of the same patient. In contrast, transform algorithms, such as FBP, can only exploit the smoothness constraints enforced by the apodization window.

An iterative reconstruction algorithm is defined by five components [Fessler, 1994],

(1) *a finite parameterization of the image,* usually represented as a discrete set of voxels,

(2) *a model of the measurement,* relating the discrete data to the image. The model is usually a linear set of equations of the type $\mathbf{p} = \mathbf{Af}$, where $\mathbf{p}$ and $\mathbf{f}$ are vectors

representing the projection and image values, and **A** is the *transition or system matrix*,

(3) *a model of noise*, i.e. of the probability distribution of the data around their expectation value,

(4) *an objective function*. This function quantifies the extent to which an image fits the data and satisfies any prescribed *a priori* constraints such as positivity and smoothness. Typical examples are the Poisson likelihood and the Gaussian likelihood, the latter of which is equivalent to the classical chi-square error,

(5) *an iterative algorithm* defining successive estimates of the image which, in principle, converge towards a solution maximizing the objective function. The specification includes a rule to decide when to stop the iteration.

The most well-known of the iterative methods is the maximum-likelihood by expectation-maximization (ML-EM) algorithm that seeks to maximize the logarithm of the Poisson likelihood objective function,

$$L(\mathbf{f}) = \sum_j \left\{ p_j \ln\left(\sum_i A_{ji} f_i \right) - \sum_i A_{ji} f_i \right\}$$

where $\mathbf{f} = \{f_i \mid i = 1,\ldots,n\}$ is a vector of the n voxel values of the image, $\mathbf{p} = \{p_j \mid j = 1,\ldots,m\}$ are the m projection values, $m = N_{x_r} \times N_\phi$ and $\mathbf{A} = \{A_{ji}\}$ is the $m \times n$ system matrix that gives the probability of a photon emitted from voxel i being detected in projection bin j. The logarithm of the likelihood objective function is maximized instead of the likelihood function itself, since the calculations are simpler and both reach their maximum for the same image. The ML-EM algorithm iteratively updates voxel values by using the EM algorithm [Shepp and Vardi, 1982],

$$f_i^{k+1} = \frac{f_i^k}{\sum_{j=1}^{m} A_{ji}} \sum_{j=1}^{m} A_{ji} \frac{p_j}{\sum_{i'=1}^{n} A_{ji'} f_{i'}^k}$$

where $\mathbf{f}^k$ is the k-th estimate of the image. One of the advantages of the ML-EM algorithm is that if the original image estimate, $\mathbf{f}^0$, is non-negative, then all subsequent estimates are also non-negative. This is a convenient method for including the *a priori* information that the reconstructed image should not contain negative values. A difficulty of statistical iterative methods such as ML-EM is the need to include regularization, similar to the need for the apodizing window function used in 2D FBP. Regularization of ML-EM is typically done by stopping after a predetermined number of cycles, possibly followed by smoothing of the image. More rigorous forms of regularization incorporate *a priori* information, although this can add to the computational load of the algorithm [Herbert and Leahy, 1989].

Iterative methods may take many cycles to converge to an acceptable solution, and each iteration essentially takes as much computation as the FBP algorithm. With the gains in computer processing speed and the development of faster iterative algorithms during the last decade, however, the additional time required for 2D iterative algorithms has become less significant.

Image Reconstruction for 3D PET

DIFFERENCES BETWEEN TWO- AND THREE-DIMENSIONAL PET IMAGING

There are two major differences between 2D and 3D PET imaging; data redundancy and spatial variance. These differences complicate 3D image reconstruction, and we will deal with them separately below. There are other differences, of course, such as the increase in scattered coincidences, but as in the previous review of 2D image reconstruction, we will assume that corrections for these effects have been applied, and that the projection data represent line-integrals through the 3D tracer as given by,

$$p(x_r, y_r, \phi, \theta) = \int_{-\infty}^{\infty} dz_r \, f(x, y, z) \tag{2.18}$$

where the 3D rotation of coordinates is given by,

$$\begin{bmatrix} x \\ y \\ z \end{bmatrix} = \begin{bmatrix} -\sin\phi & -\cos\phi\sin\theta & \cos\phi\cos\theta \\ \cos\phi & -\sin\phi\sin\theta & \sin\phi\cos\theta \\ 0 & \cos\theta & \sin\theta \end{bmatrix} \begin{bmatrix} x_r \\ y_r \\ z_r \end{bmatrix} \tag{2.19}$$

To illustrate the data redundancy of 3D PET imaging, consider that in normal 2D PET imaging of a volume (using septa), we have sufficient information to reconstruct the tracer distribution. In performing 3D imaging of the same volume, we collect a super-set of the 2D data, therefore the additional data must consist of redundant information. The key point of 3D PET imaging is that the collection of this redundant information along the additional LORs, if used properly, can improve image SNR by reducing statistical noise.

The shift variance of 3D PET can be understood by considering fig. 2.16, which illustrates how a projection is *truncated* due to the finite axial extent of the scanner. To develop the theory and algorithms required to reconstruct the tracer distribution, we will need to assume that $p(x_r, y_r, \phi, \theta)$ is known for all (x_r, y_r). In other words, we need to measure all LORs parallel to $\hat{\mathbf{z}}_r = (\cos\phi\cos\theta, \sin\phi\cos\theta, \sin\theta)$ (defined in fig. 2.3) and crossing the region D_f, where D_f is the support of the object, that is, where $f(\mathbf{x}) \neq 0$. If the projections are not truncated, they are said to be *complete.* If all projections were complete, the sensitivity of the scanner would be independent of the position in the field-of-view and the reconstruction problem would be stationary (*shift-invariant*) and could be solved using standard Fourier deconvolution techniques. The 2D reconstruction problem, with a multi-ring scanner operated with the septa extended, is shift-invariant provided small effects such as the parallax error are neglected or corrected. In contrast, the 3D problem is not shift-invariant because the solid angle subtended by the scanner decreases when one moves away from the center of the field-of-view (FOV) along the scanner axis. Thus, as can be seen from fig. 2.16, a 2D projection measured by a cylindrical scanner is complete only when $|\theta| < \Theta_c$, where Θ_c depends on the size of the region D_f [2] relative to the scanner dimensions.

---

[2]For the value of Θ_C indicated in fig. 2.16, the allowable size of the region D_f is actually slightly larger than the cylindrical FOV shown, but has a more complicated shape.

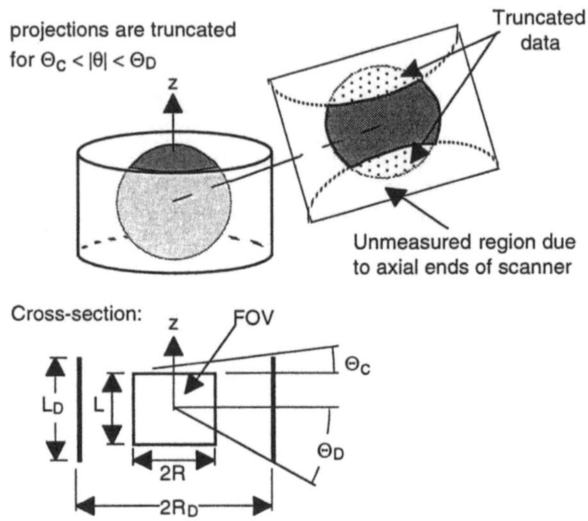

Figure 2.16 Illustration of the region of complete data acquisition for a 3D PET scanner.

Usually, D_f extends axially beyond the FOV of the scanner, (that is L > L_D in fig. 2.16) and Θ_c is then equal to zero. In such a case, the only complete projections are those that correspond to ring differences $\Delta r = 0$ and $\Delta r = \pm 1$. Truncation increases the complexity of the reconstruction because filtered-backprojection, being based on Fourier deconvolution, cannot be applied to incomplete data. The standard solution to this difficulty consists of first estimating the truncated data to obtain a set of complete 2D projections along all directions

$$\hat{\mathbf{z}}_r(\phi,\theta) = (\cos\phi\cos\theta, \sin\phi\cos\theta, \sin\theta), \quad 0 \le \phi < \pi, \quad |\theta| \le \Theta \tag{2.20}$$

where the estimation step and the choice of $\Theta, (\Theta_c \le \Theta \le \Theta_D)$ is discussed after the next section. We next describe the second step, the reconstruction of *f(x,y,z)* from complete projections.

3D FBP FOR COMPLETE 2D PARALLEL PROJECTIONS

This section describes the theory and algorithms required to reconstruct the tracer distribution *f(x,y,z)* from 3D PET data consisting of a set of 2D parallel-projections. We assume in this section that $p(x_r, y_r, \phi, \theta)$ is known for $0 \le \phi < \pi, |\theta| \le \Theta$ and for all (x_r, y_r), that is, that all projections are complete.

The 3D central-section theorem. The cornerstone of 3D image reconstruction is the 3D central-section theorem , which generalizes the 2D central-section theorem.

Define first the 3D Fourier transform of the image as,

$$F(\upsilon_x,\upsilon_y,\upsilon_z)=\int_{-\infty}^{+\infty}dx\int_{-\infty}^{+\infty}dy\int_{-\infty}^{+\infty}dz\,e^{-2\pi i(x\upsilon_x+y\upsilon_y+z\upsilon_z)}f(x,y,z) \tag{2.21}$$

and also define the 2D Fourier transform with respect to the first two coordinates of a parallel projection perpendicular to $\hat{\mathbf{z}}_r(\phi,\theta)$:

$$P(\upsilon_{xr},\upsilon_{yr},\phi,\theta)=\int_{-\infty}^{+\infty}dx_r\int_{-\infty}^{+\infty}dy_r\,e^{-2\pi i(x_r\upsilon_{xr}+y_r\upsilon_{yr})}p(x_r,y_r,\phi,\theta) \tag{2.22}$$

Note that the integral in equation 2.22 is over the entire region where $p(x_r,y_r,\phi,\theta)\neq 0$ and therefore the Fourier transform can not be calculated from truncated projections. The 3D central-section theorem is illustrated in fig. 2.17, and relates the Fourier transform of the image and data as:

$$P(\upsilon_{xr},\upsilon_{yr},\phi,\theta)=F(\upsilon_x,\upsilon_y,\upsilon_z)\big|_{\upsilon_{zr}=0} \tag{2.23}$$

where the frequency coordinates in the image and projection spaces are related by the same rotation matrix as in equation 2.19:

$$\begin{bmatrix}\upsilon_x\\ \upsilon_y\\ \upsilon_z\end{bmatrix}=\begin{bmatrix}-\sin\phi & -\cos\phi\sin\theta & \cos\phi\cos\theta\\ \cos\phi & -\sin\phi\sin\theta & \sin\phi\cos\theta\\ 0 & \cos\theta & \sin\theta\end{bmatrix}\begin{bmatrix}\upsilon_{xr}\\ \upsilon_{yr}\\ \upsilon_{zr}\end{bmatrix} \tag{2.24}$$

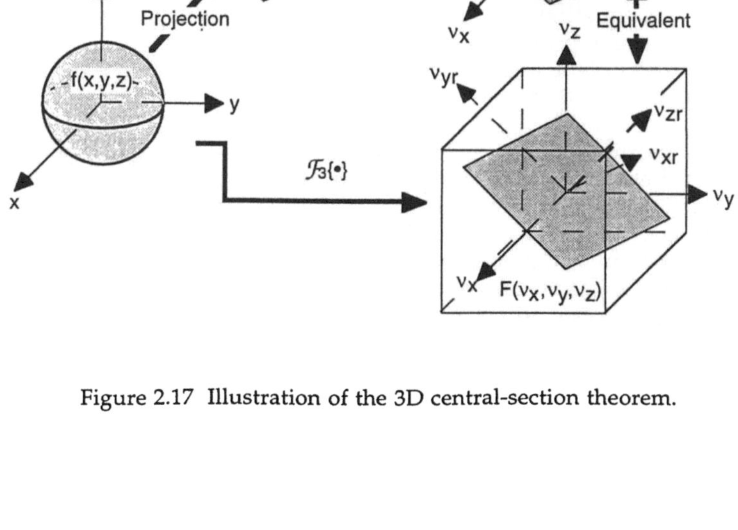

Figure 2.17 Illustration of the 3D central-section theorem.

Given a 2D projection perpendicular to $\hat{\mathbf{z}}_r(\phi,\theta)$, equation 2.23 can serve to calculate the 3D Fourier transform of the image for any frequency $(\upsilon_x, \upsilon_y, \upsilon_z)$ contained in the plane $\upsilon_{zr} = 0$, as defined by equation 2.24. As can easily be seen, any such frequency is orthogonal to the projection direction $\hat{\mathbf{z}}_r(\phi,\theta)$. Geometrically, this means that a 2D parallel projection allows to recover $F(\upsilon_x, \upsilon_y, \upsilon_z)$ on a plane containing the origin and orthogonal to $\hat{\mathbf{z}}_r(\phi,\theta)$ in the 3D image frequency space. We next describe how reconstruction algorithms are obtained from this property.

The redundancy of the 3D data. Consider first a 2D acquisition where $p(x_r, y_r, \phi, \theta)$ is measured only for $\theta = 0$. For each ϕ, the 3D central-section theorem yields $F(\upsilon_x, \upsilon_y, \upsilon_z)$ on a plane containing the υ_z axis. When the azimuthal angle ϕ varies over its range $[0,\pi)$ that plane rotates around the υ_z axis and sweeps the entire 3D frequency space, allowing the whole 3D Fourier transform of $f(x,y,z)$, and hence the image itself, to be reconstructed. This is illustrated in fig. 2.18.

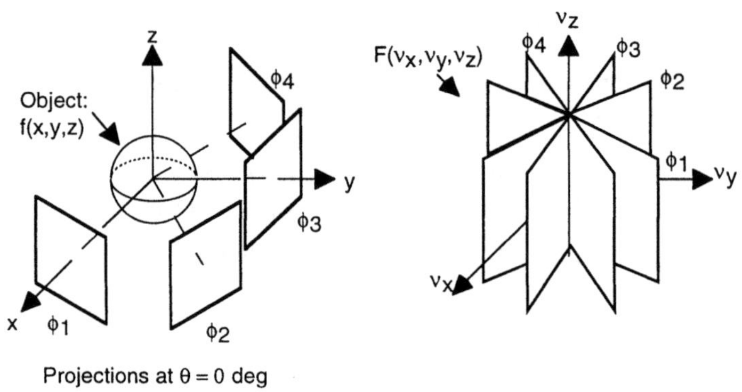

Figure 2.18 Illustration of how the 3D central-section can be used to reconstruct $F(\upsilon_x, \upsilon_y, \upsilon_z)$ from $p(x_r, y_r, \phi, \theta)$ using only projections with $\theta = 0$.

As can be seen from equation 2.24, in this 2D case, a given frequency $(\upsilon_x, \upsilon_y, \upsilon_z)$ can be retrieved from a single projection, defined by $\phi = \arctan(-\upsilon_x/\upsilon_y)$. The 2D data, therefore, are not redundant, and this results in the ramp filter being unique (up to the choice of the regularizing window).

To understand the sampling of the 3D Fourier transform in the more general case of 3D PET imaging, it is helpful to use the notation introduced by Orlov in his seminal papers on 3D reconstruction in electron microscopy [Orlov, 1976; Orlov, 1976]. As shown in fig. 2.19(a), the orientation of a single 2D projection plane can be described by the location of the end point of the unit vector $\hat{\mathbf{z}}_r(\phi,\theta)$, on the unit sphere. The set of such end-points is labeled Ω, as is shown in fig. 2.19(b) for the same single projection in fig. 2.19(a). The set Ω_0 corresponding to the projections in fig. 2.18 is shown in fig. 2.19(c), while 2.19(d) shows Ω_Θ for general 3D imaging. It is worth noting that Orlov's theorem states that a 3D data set is complete if there is no unit great circle that does not intersect Ω.

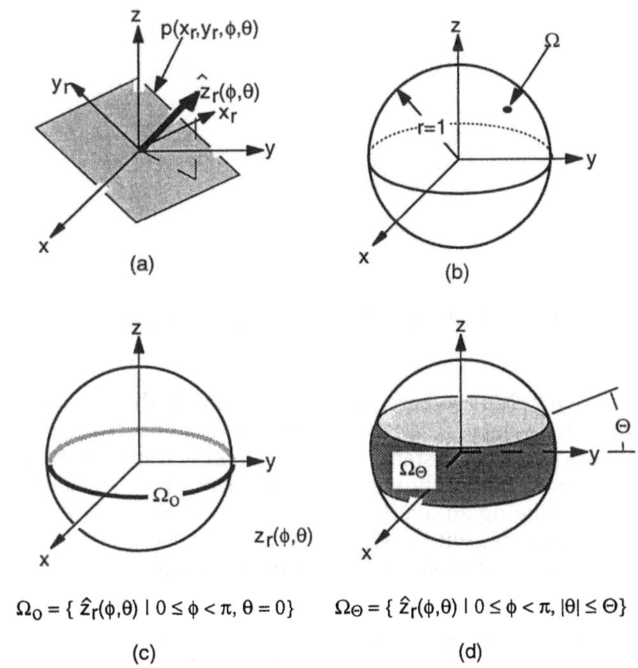

Figure 2.19 Orlov Spheres for different scanning geometries.

Consider now the 3D data set of equation 2.18. The value of the 3D Fourier transform of the image at a frequency $\overline{\upsilon}=(\upsilon_x,\upsilon_y,\upsilon_z)$ can be calculated by applying the 3D central-section theorem to any measured 2D projection such that $\hat{\mathbf{z}}_r(\phi,\theta)$ is orthogonal to $\overline{\upsilon}$:

$$\overline{\upsilon}\cdot\hat{z}_r(\phi,\theta)=\upsilon_x\cos\phi\cos\theta+\upsilon_y\sin\phi\cos\theta+\upsilon_z\sin\theta=0 \tag{2.25}$$

In general this equation has a continuum of solutions within the measured range $0\le\phi<\pi$, $|\theta|\le\Theta$ and the 3D data are therefore redundant. If the frequency is represented using polar coordinates (υ,α,ψ) defined as:

$$\overline{\upsilon}=(\upsilon_x,\upsilon_y,\upsilon_z)=(\upsilon\cos\alpha\cos\psi,\upsilon\sin\alpha\cos\psi,\upsilon\sin\psi) \tag{2.26}$$

equation 2.25 becomes:

$$\cos(\phi-\alpha)=-\tan\psi\tan\theta,\ \text{for}\ \upsilon\neq 0 \tag{2.27}$$

This equation has a solution for ϕ if and only if $|\sin\theta|\le|\cos\psi|$. Hence $F(\overline{\upsilon})$ can be calculated using any projection (ϕ,θ) with $\theta\in[-\Theta_{\lim},+\Theta_{\lim}]$ and ϕ given by the solution of equation 2.27, where the angle $\Theta_{\lim}$ is defined by:

$$\Theta_{\lim}=\begin{cases}\Theta, & \cos\psi>\sin\Theta\\ \pi/2-\psi, & \cos\psi\le\sin\Theta\end{cases} \tag{2.28}$$

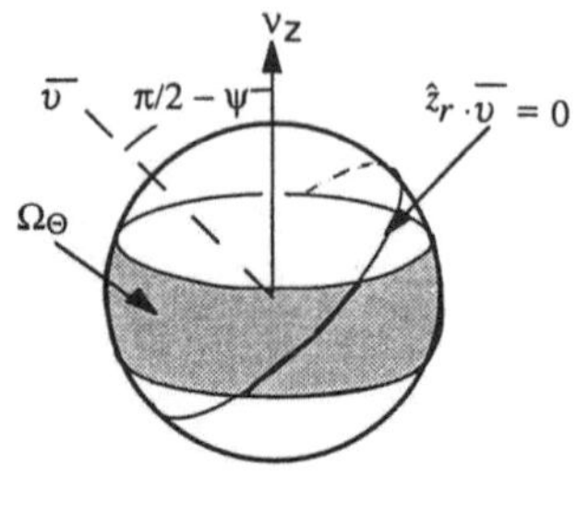

Figure 2.20 Coordinates for the filter equation.

This is illustrated in fig. 2.20, where the intersection of this set with the great circle orthogonal to some frequency $\overline{\upsilon}$ is the set of projections from which $F(\overline{\upsilon})$ can be obtained. If the data were consistent, all these independent estimates of $F(\overline{\upsilon})$ would be equal. In the presence of noise, however, the data are not consistent and an optimal SNR is obtained by averaging all available estimates of $F(\overline{\upsilon})$. The standard approach involves a weighted average, with a weighting factor $\cos\theta/\sqrt{\cos^2\psi-\sin^2\theta}$, which can be shown to provide a uniform solid angle sampling in (ϕ,θ):

$$F(\overline{\upsilon}) = H(\Theta,\psi)\int_{-\Theta_{\lim}}^{+\Theta_{\lim}} d\theta \frac{2\cos\theta}{\sqrt{\cos^2\psi-\sin^2\theta}} P(\upsilon_{xr},\upsilon_{yr},\phi,\theta) \tag{2.29}$$

where $\Theta_{\lim}$ is given by equation 2.28, and $H(\Theta,\psi)$ is the normalization factor which ensures that $F\equiv 1$ if $P\equiv 1$:

$$\frac{1}{H(\Theta,\psi)} = \int_{-\Theta_{\lim}}^{+\Theta_{\lim}} d\theta \frac{2\cos\theta}{\sqrt{\cos^2\psi-\sin^2\theta}} = \begin{cases} 2\pi & \cos\psi \le \sin\Theta \\ 4\arcsin\left(\dfrac{\sin\Theta}{\cos\psi}\right) & \cos\psi > \sin\Theta \end{cases} \tag{2.30}$$

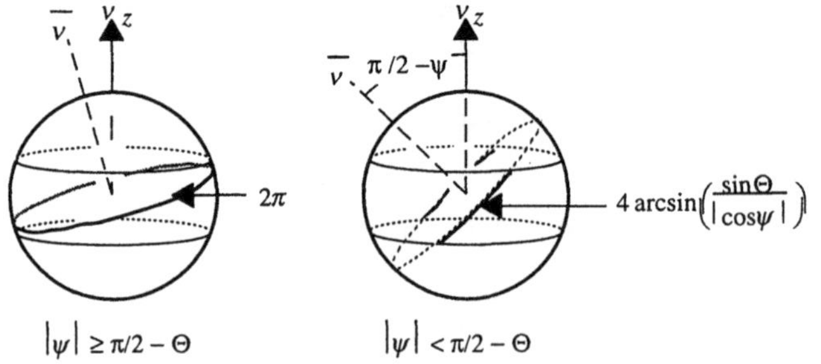

Figure 2.21 The normalizing arc lengths corresponding to the sampling by projections in the two different regions in the Fourier transform of the object.

This is illustrated in fig. 2.21, which shows the two different regions in frequency space and the arc lengths corresponding to the normalizing factors for the sampling of the 3D Fourier transform.

A direct implementation of equation 2.29 leads to the 3D *direct Fourier reconstruction algorithm*, which is analogous to the 2D direct Fourier reconstruction algorithm. This algorithm proceeds in two steps. First, for each 3D frequency, equation 2.29 is used to estimate $F(\overline{\upsilon})$ from the 2D Fourier transform of the projection data. Then, the image is recovered by inverse 3D Fourier transform. This algorithm makes extensive use of the Fast Fourier Transform (FFT) but this advantage is largely offset by the need for a rather complicated interpolation in frequency space. This interpolation is necessary because the FFT generates the 2D Fourier transform of a projection on a rectangular grid in $(\upsilon_{xr}, \upsilon_{yr})$, and this grid is not mapped by equation 2.24 onto the cubic grid $(\upsilon_x, \upsilon_y, \upsilon_z)$ required for the inverse 3D FFT. A similar problem occurs in 2D (fig. 2.13), and, both in 2D and in 3D, FBP algorithms are normally preferred to direct Fourier reconstruction.

The 3D filtered-backprojection algorithm. The standard method to reconstruct 3D PET data is the *3D filtered-backprojection* (3D FBP) algorithm. This algorithm is derived by calculating analytically the inverse 3D Fourier transform of equation 2.29 to avoid interpolations in frequency space. Apart from the higher dimension, 3D FBP algorithm is similar to 2D FBP:

(1) Filtering of projections for each (ϕ, θ):

1.1 calculate the 2D Fourier transform $P(\upsilon_{xr}, \upsilon_{yr}, \phi, \theta)$, using equation 2.22,

1.2 multiply by a 2D filter H_C, and a 2D window W, both described below:

$$P^F(\upsilon_{xr}, \upsilon_{yr}, \phi, \theta) = P(\upsilon_{xr}, \upsilon_{yr}, \phi, \theta)\, H_C(\upsilon_{xr}, \upsilon_{yr}, \theta)\, W(\upsilon_{xr}, \upsilon_{yr}) \tag{2.31}$$

1.3 take the inverse 2D Fourier transform to get a filtered projection,

$$p^F(x_r, y_r, \phi, \theta) = \int_{-\infty}^{+\infty} d\upsilon_{xr} \int_{-\infty}^{+\infty} d\upsilon_{yr}\, e^{2\pi i(x_r \upsilon_{xr} + y_r \upsilon_{yr})} P^F(\upsilon_{xr}, \upsilon_{yr}, \phi, \theta)$$

(2) 3D backprojection of the filtered projections:

$$f(x,y,z) = f(x,y,z) + (\cos\theta\, \Delta\theta\, \Delta\phi)\, p^F(x_r, y_r, \phi, \theta) \tag{2.32}$$

(3) repeat steps 1-2 for each $\phi: 0 \le \phi < \pi$

(4) repeat steps 1-3 for each $\theta: -\Theta \le \theta < \Theta$

In equation 2.32 x_r and y_r are obtained by solving equation 2.19 with the requirement that the LOR defined by (x_r, y_r, ϕ, θ) contains the point (x, y, z).

The 2D filter H_C, in equation 2.31 is the filter derived by Colsher [Colsher, 1980]. This filter properly takes into account the redundancy of the data, and is related to the normalization factor for the weighted average in equation 2.29 by:

$$H_C(\upsilon_{xr}, \upsilon_{yr}, \theta) = \sqrt{\upsilon_{xr}^2 + \upsilon_{yr}^2}\, H(\Theta, \psi) \tag{2.33}$$

where $H(\Theta,\psi)$ is given by equation 2.30, and the co-polar angle ψ of the 3D frequency can be written in terms of the projection frequency υ_{xr} and υ_{yr} using equation 2.24:

$$\tan^2\psi = \frac{\upsilon_{yr}^2\cos^2\theta}{\upsilon_{xr}^2+\upsilon_{yr}^2\sin^2\theta} \tag{2.34}$$

The angular and radial dependencies of Colsher's filter are clearly separated in equation 2.33. The radial factor is the modulus of the frequency, $\sqrt{\upsilon_{xr}^2+\upsilon_{yr}^2}$, and is similar to the ramp filter $|\upsilon|$ in 2D FBP. As will be seen in the last section of this chapter, this property results in the 2D and 3D FBP algorithms having similar noise properties.

The *apodization window* $W(\upsilon_{xr},\upsilon_{yr})$ in equation 2.31 is designed to restrict the noise amplification by Colsher's filter. As in 2D image reconstruction, the choice of W depends on the noise level and is usually empirically determined. Typically one uses a Hamming window (equation 2.16) with an appropriate cut-off frequency, either in the form of a Cartesian product $W_H(\upsilon_{xr})W_H(\upsilon_{yr})$ or as a radially symmetrical window $W_H(\sqrt{\upsilon_{xr}^2+\upsilon_{yr}^2})$. The former choice allows to select the same apodization as in a 2D reconstruction, while the latter choice is consistent with the 3D nature of the problem.

A few remarks are in order concerning the discrete implementation of the 3D FBP algorithm. In the *filtering step*, a 2D projection is first included in a larger matrix, the dimensions of which (both in x_r and y_r) are typically twice the dimensions of the original data. This *zero-padding* technique aims at avoiding circular convolution artifacts. The 2D FFT of the padded data is obtained on a square grid $(\upsilon_{xr},\upsilon_{yr})$, and each frequency sample $P(\upsilon_{xr},\upsilon_{yr},\phi,\theta)$ is multiplied by the corresponding element of a digital 2D filter. This digital filter can be built by simply sampling the continuous filter function (the apodized filter of Colsher), but this method may generate artifacts, chiefly appearing as a small shift in the DC level. A more accurate filter can be obtained using the same approach as in 2D tomography: first the convolution kernel is calculated as the continuous inverse Fourier transform of the analytical filter, this kernel is then discretized and the digital filter is finally obtained by taking the FFT of the kernel. A variation of this technique for Colsher's filter has been described by Stearns [Stearns et al., 1994].

The discrete implementation of the *3D backprojection* is straightforward: the integrals over θ and ϕ in equation 2.32 are approximated by means of trapezoidal quadratures and a voxel driven backprojection (where the center of each voxel is forward-projected onto the 2D (x_r,y_r)plane) is then used with bilinear interpolation in the (x_r,y_r) plane. The major problem with 3D backprojection, especially for modern scanners, is that as many as 20 million LORs must be backprojected. Besides the use of high speed hardware (described in chapter 5), various software methods have been proposed to speed up 3D backprojection, including incremental backprojection and the exploitation of geometrical symmetries [Egger, 1996]. A last point of interest concerning the implementation of the backprojection is the choice of the integration variables. The parallel projections are sometimes parameterized using the ring-difference Δr (fig. 2.10) instead of the co-polar angle θ. In this case, the integration variable in the backprojection integral must be modified, and a Jacobian $|d\theta/d\Delta r|$ must be included. When Θ is small, however, the Jacobian is to a good approximation constant.

THE 3D REPROJECTION ALGORITHM.

What is truncation and how does it influence reconstruction? Previously we saw how the image *f(x,y,z)* was reconstructed from 2D parallel projections $p(x_r, y_r, \phi, \theta)$ measured for a set of directions $\Omega_\Theta = \{(\theta,\phi) \mid 0 \le \phi < \pi, |\theta| \le \Theta\}$. The 3D FBP algorithm was derived assuming complete projections such that, for each direction $\hat{\mathbf{z}}_r(\theta,\phi) \in \Omega$, $p(x_r, y_r, \phi, \theta)$ is measured for all $(x_r, y_r) \in D_p$, where D_p is the support of the projection of the object. For instance, if $f(x,y,z) \neq 0$ in a cylinder with the same length L_D as the scanner and a radius $R < R_D$, then the support of the orthogonal projection of the cylinder along a direction $\hat{\mathbf{z}}_r(\phi,\theta)$ is:

$$D_p = \left\{ (x_r, y_r) \middle| \, |x_r| < R, \, |y_r| < \frac{L_D}{2\cos\theta} + |\sin\theta| \sqrt{R^2 - x_r^2} \right\} \tag{2.35}$$

Note that D_p is independent of ϕ due to the rotational symmetry of the scanner. A cylindrical scanner, however, measures the projection $p(x_r, y_r, \phi, \theta)$ in a region:

$$M_p = \left\{ (x_r, y_r) \middle| \, |x_r| < R_D, \, |y_r| < \frac{L_D}{2\cos\theta} - |\sin\theta| \sqrt{R_D^2 - x_r^2} \right\} \tag{2.36}$$

Note that the measured y_r range at the center of the field of view $(x_r = 0)$ decreases with increasing θ and vanishes when $|\theta| = \Theta_D$. As shown in fig. 2.16, for $\theta \neq 0$, the measured region M_p does not contain the projection of the object, D_p, and hence the projection is truncated. Applying 3D FBP to truncated projections results in severe artifacts, which essentially reflect the drop of the scanner sensitivity when moving from the center $(z = 0)$ towards the edge of the field-of-view $(z = \pm L_D / 2)$. Unfortunately, these truncation artifacts cannot be corrected by simply dividing in each point the FBP reconstruction by the sensitivity in that point. This can be understood by rewriting the filtering equation 2.31 as a 2D convolution:

$$p^F(x_r, y_r, \phi, \theta) = \iint_{D_p} dx_r' \, dy_r' \, h_C(x_r - x_r', y_r - y_r', \phi, \theta) p(x_r', y_r', \phi, \theta) \tag{2.37}$$

where the convolution kernel $h_C(x_r, y_r, \phi, \theta)$, is the inverse 2D Fourier transform of the apodized Colsher's filter:

$$h_C(x_r, y_r, \phi, \theta) = \int_{-\infty}^{+\infty} d\upsilon_{xr} \int_{-\infty}^{+\infty} d\upsilon_{yr} \, e^{2\pi i (x_r \upsilon_{xr} + y_r \upsilon_{yr})} H_C(\upsilon_{xr}, \upsilon_{yr}, \theta) W(\upsilon_{xr}, \upsilon_{yr}) \tag{2.38}$$

One can show that $h(x_r, y_r, \phi, \theta)$ is non zero for all (x_r, y_r) and therefore the value of the filtered projection $p^F(x_r, y_r, \phi, \theta)$ in any point (x_r, y_r) depends on the value of $p(x_r', y_r', \phi, \theta)$ for all $(x_r', y_r') \in D_p$. This property is related to the *non-local* character of 2D and 3D tomographic reconstructions[3]: the value of the image in some point $\mathbf{x}$ cannot be reconstructed using only the LORs which cross some small neighborhood of $\mathbf{x}$.

The 3DRP algorithm. The 3D reprojection (3DRP) algorithm [Kinahan and Rogers, 1989] is the standard method used to reconstruct truncated 3D PET data. In the 3DRP

---

[3]Local tomographic reconstruction is possible but yields only non-quantitative images, which provide information over the discontinuities of *f*(**x**), that is, on the boundaries between regions where the tracer concentration varies smoothly.

method, complete 2D projections are obtained by estimating $p(x_r, y_r, \phi, \theta)$ in the unmeasured region $\{(x_r, y_r) \mid (x_r, y_r) \in D_p, (x_r, y_r) \notin M_p\}$. Filtered-backprojection can then be applied to the completed projections, which are partly measured and partly synthesized. The truncated data are estimated by calculating line integrals (equation 2.18) of an image $f_{2D}(x, y, z)$ reconstructed from the 2D projections with $\theta = 0$, i.e. from the data subset corresponding to a 2D acquisition. These projections are not truncated, as can be seen by taking $\theta = 0$ in equations 2.35 and 2.36, and $f_{2D}(x, y, z)$ can thus be reconstructed using standard 2D FBP. In the absence of noise, this 2D reconstruction would be accurate and thus $f_{2D}(x, y, z)$ is an unbiased estimator of the true image. This estimator, however, has more variance than the final 3D reconstruction since it only incorporates a subset of the data.

In practice, the 2D projections are measured for discrete values of the angle θ, corresponding to integer values of the ring difference index (fig. 2.10). The implementation of the 3DRP algorithm requires the specification of the data subset to be used to reconstruct $f_{2D}(x, y, z)$. The minimum subset consists of the coincidences with ring differences $\Delta r = 0$ and $\Delta r = \pm 1$, which are sufficient to reconstruct the whole field-of-view. To improve the statistical accuracy of the estimated image one usually includes coincidences with larger values of Δr, e.g. $|\Delta r| \leq 5$, following the standard 2D reconstruction procedure applied when the scanner is operated with the septa extended. The choice of the maximum value of Δr entails a compromise between systematic and statistical errors for $f_{2D}(x, y, z)$. Empirically, however, experience has shown that the quality of the final image $f(x,y,z)$, is not strongly dependent on the maximum value of Δr used to estimate $f_{2D}(x, y, z)$.

The steps of the 3DRP algorithm are (fig. 2.22):

(1) extract the 2D data from the full data set for 2D reconstruction,

(2) reconstruct a first image estimate $f_{2D}(x, y, z)$ by applying, for each slice z, 2D FBP,

(3) for each projection (ϕ, θ), with $0 \leq \phi < \pi$ and $|\theta| \leq \Theta$

(3.1) estimate the truncated data as in equation 2.18:

$$p(x_r, y_r, \phi, \theta) = \int_{-\infty}^{+\infty} dz_r\, f_{2D}(x, y, z), \quad \{(x_r, y_r) | (x_r, y_r) \in D_p, (x_r, y_r) \notin M_p\}$$

(3.2) merge the estimated and measured data,

- the subsequent steps correspond to the 3D FBP method:

(3.3) take the 2D FFT to get $P(\upsilon_{xr}, \upsilon_{yr}, \phi, \theta)$,

(3.4) multiply by the apodized Colsher's filter $H_C(\upsilon_{xr}, \upsilon_{yr}, \theta) W(\upsilon_{xr}, \upsilon_{yr})$,

(3.5) take the inverse 2D FFT to get $p^F(x_r, y_r, \phi, \theta)$,

(3.6) backproject through the 3D image volume according to equation 2.32.

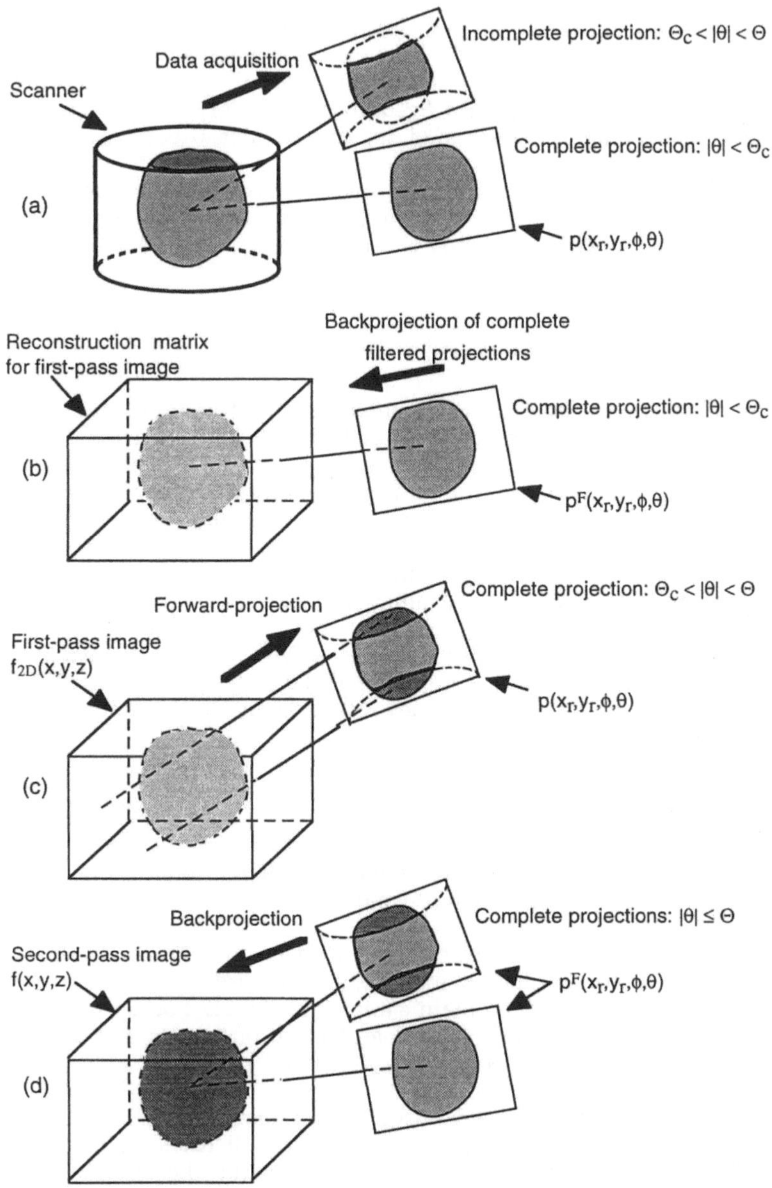

Figure 2.22 The 3DRP algorithm. (a) Collection of truncated projections by the PET scanner. (b) Reconstruction of the first-pass image $f_{2D}(x, y, z)$ using the complete projection data $|\theta| \leq \Theta_C$. (c) Estimation of the truncated projection data by forward projection through the first-pass image. (d) Reconstruction of the second-pass image $f(x,y,z)$, using the complete projection set. Note that for step (b), in practice $\Theta_C = 0$.

The maximum value of θ incorporated in the reconstruction, Θ, is usually smaller than the scanner aperture $\Theta_D = \arctan(L_D/2R_D)$. This choice is made since when $|\theta| \approx \Theta_D$, the measured region M_p becomes much smaller than the required region D_p, as can be seen from equations 2.35 and 2.36 and from fig. 2.16. Thus, for large $|\theta|$, the completed projection data consists mainly of estimated, rather than measured, data.

Reducing the value of Θ saves significant computation without sacrificing much sensitivity, as shown below. A maximum ring difference of 17 is typical for a 24 ring scanner, corresponding to Θ = 12 degrees. In this case, a full 93% of the data are incorporated in the reconstruction.

Alternative 3D Reconstruction Methods.

The 3DRP algorithm is used by most PET centers involved in routine 3D acquisition. The considerable experience accumulated since 1990 has confirmed the accuracy and robustness of this algorithm. Several alternative algorithms have been proposed, either to decrease the reconstruction time or to improve image quality. Three of these algorithms described below, the single-slice rebinning, the multi-slice rebinning, and the Fourier rebinning algorithms, are implemented in the software provided with some commercial scanners. The other algorithms described below are currently under development and still await a thorough evaluation.

Three types of methods will be considered: those derived from exact *analytic* inversion formula as described above, those that *rebin* the 3D data onto an ordinary 2D data set, and finally those based on *iterative* techniques. More details on these algorithms can be found in the noted references.

ANALYTIC METHODS.

Analytic, or *transform*, algorithms are obtained by discretizing exact inversion formulae for equation 2.18. Algorithms in this class, such as the 3DRP algorithm, would provide exact reconstructions in the absence of noise and of discretization errors.

The *direct Fourier reconstruction* algorithm, developed by Stearns et al [Stearns et al., 1990], is faster than 3DRP. because it makes extensive use of the FFT. However, a complex interpolation is required to obtain samples of the 3D Fourier transform of the image on a cubic grid from the available samples located on a square grid in an oblique central plane orthogonal to the projection direction $\hat{\mathbf{z}}_r(\phi,\theta)$.

Accurate interpolation methods based on gridding [Stearns et al., 1990] have been proposed, but restrict the speed up factor with respect to 3DRP to about 2. Note that the direct Fourier method requires complete projections, and the truncated data must therefore be estimated as in the 3DRP algorithm.

The 3DRP algorithm is based on the filter of Colsher, equation 2.30, which has optimal noise properties under fairly general conditions. Owing to the redundancy of the 3D data, a large number of other filters can be derived by modifying the weighting factor in the weighted average (equation 2.29). This freedom can be exploited to define filters which facilitate numerical implementation.

One example is the *Favor* algorithm [Defrise et al., 1991], which is a 3D FBP algorithm with the filter of Colsher replaced by another exact filter chosen in such a way that it reduces for all truncated projections (in practice, for $|\theta| > \Theta_c$) to the 1D ramp filter along the x_r axis:

$$H_{Favor}(\nu_{xr}, \nu_{yr}, \theta) = |\nu_{xr}|, \text{ for } |\theta| > \Theta_c \tag{2.39}$$

The form of the filter for $|\theta| \leq \Theta_c$ can be found in [Defrise et al., 1991]. The advantage of this choice is that the filtered projections can be calculated within the measured region M_p using only measured data, and consequently the truncated data need no longer be calculated by forward projection as in the 3DRP algorithm. The Favor algorithm is thus about 50% faster than the 3DRP method [Egger, 1996].

REBINNING METHODS.

The time required to reconstruct 3D data with the 3DRP algorithm is more than an order of magnitude longer than the time needed to reconstruct 2D data acquired with septa. This is due to the considerable increase of the number of LORs to be backprojected. The extended memory needed to store the 3D data is another drawback of 3D acquisition.

A rebinning algorithm is defined as an algorithm which, starting from the 3D data, estimates a 2D data set containing one sinogram for each transverse slice z:

$$s(x_r, \phi, z, \Delta r) \Rightarrow s_{2D}(x_r, \phi, z) \tag{2.40}$$

where we have assumed that the 3D data are histogrammed as oblique sinograms. The rebinning process is illustrated in fig. 2.23.

Recall that $z = (r_1 + r_2)/2$ and $\Delta r = r_1 - r_2$ where r_1 and r_2 are the axial coordinates of the two rings in coincidence. Rebinning reduces image reconstruction to a 2D slice by slice reconstruction, which results in a dramatic speed up, provided of course the rebinning procedure itself is fast. An added advantage of rebinning algorithms is that they achieve at the same time an important data compression. With a N_R-ring scanner the 3D data contain N_R^2 sinograms whereas the 2D data contain usually $2N_R - 1$ sinograms, and the data compression factor is approximately $N_R/2$. The only shortcoming of the rebinning algorithms is that they are approximate and the type of studies to which they can be applied must be carefully controlled. A practical rebinning algorithm should be:

- fast ,
- accurate,
- as stable with respect to noise as a true 3D reconstruction method.

Note the importance of this last requirement. Noise-free 3D PET data are redundant in the sense that the sinograms with $\Delta r = 0, \pm 1$ are sufficient for an exact reconstruction. Hence, without the last requirement, rebinning could be achieved trivially by extracting from the 3D data the sinograms with $\Delta r = 0, \pm 1$. While valid for noise-free data, this approach would not take advantage of the increased sensitivity allowed by a 3D acquisition. An optimal signal-to-noise ratio can be obtained only if the rebinning method incorporates the whole 3D data, as does the 3DRP algorithm.

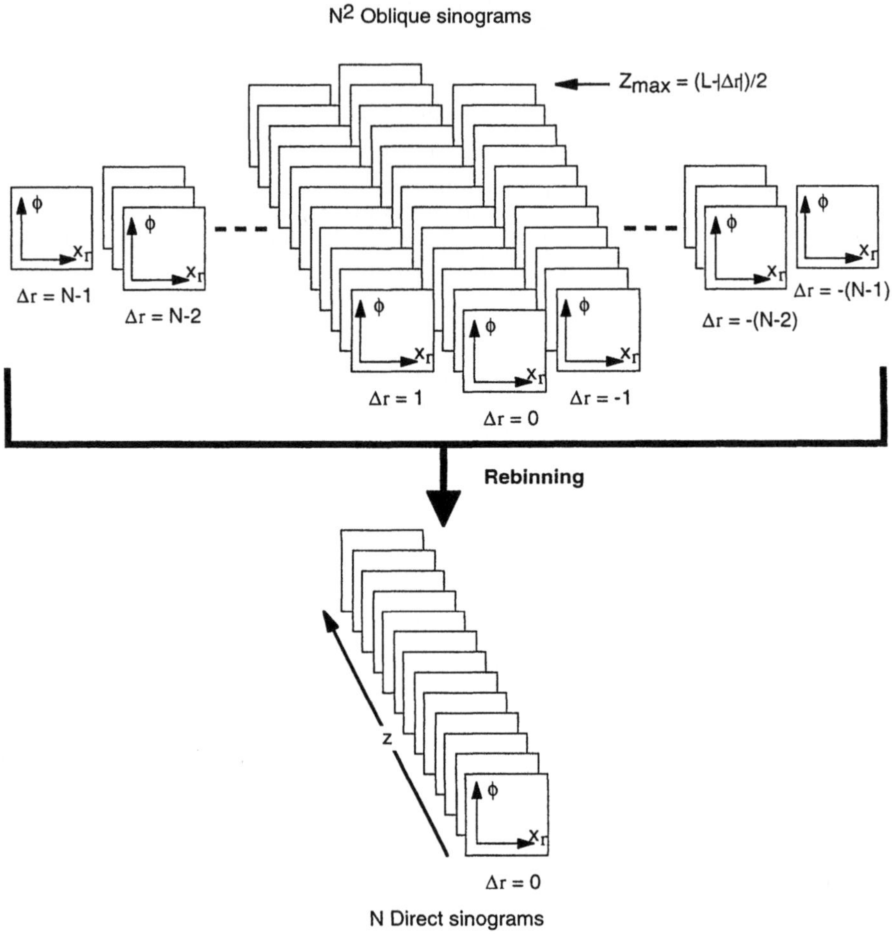

Figure 2.23 Illustration of rebinning process compressing full 3D set of oblique sinograms from a N-ring scanner into a smaller number of direct 2D sinograms.

The simplest method is the *single-slice rebinning* algorithm (SSRB) [Daube-Witherspoon and Muehllehner, 1987] which extends to 3D the standard method used to produce a set of direct-plane and cross-plane sinograms from data acquired in 2D mode. Thus, as is shown in fig. 2.24, the angle θ between an oblique LOR and the transaxial plane is neglected, and the LOR is rebinned into the transverse slice $z = (r_1 + r_2)/2$ located mid-way axially between the two detectors in coincidence.

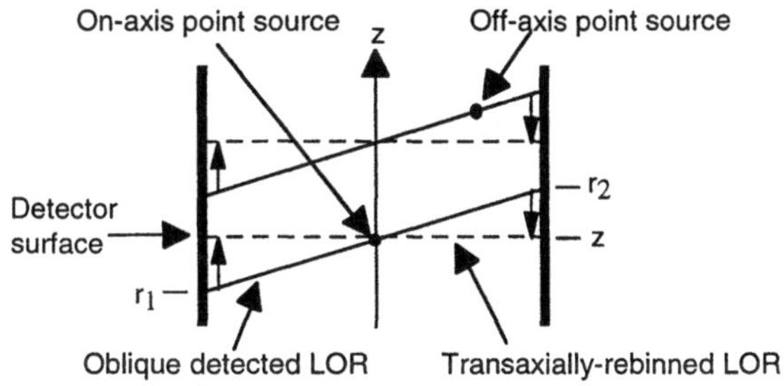

Figure 2.24 Illustration of the Single-Slice Rebinning (SSRB) method. The true oblique LORs (solid lines) are assigned to their mid-plane (dotted lines), thus distorting off-axis point sources.

In this way, the rebinned sinograms are built by averaging the 3D sinograms as:

$$s_{2D}(x_r,\phi,z)=\frac{1}{2\Delta r_{max}(z)}\int_{-\Delta r_{max}(z)}^{+\Delta r_{max}(z)} d\Delta r\, s(x_r,\phi,z,\Delta r) \tag{2.41}$$

where $\Delta r_{max}(z)$ is the maximum ring difference available for the slice at axial position z. Fig. 2.24 illustrates the fact that the accuracy of the SSRB method is good only provided the tracer is concentrated close to the axis of the scanner. Thus, accurate SSRB reconstructions have been obtained with the 16 ring ECAT 953B for receptor studies involving the human basal ganglia [Sossi et al., 1994]. For FDG brain imaging, the diameter of the transaxial FOV is larger, and larger distortions could be expected with the SSRB algorithm, especially when the brain is not well centered in the field-of-view. Even in this case, the differences with images obtained with the 3DRP algorithm are often minor because the axial aperture of many current PET scanners does not exceed 10 degrees. Other applications, however, such as whole body imaging, or brain imaging with wide aperture scanners require either exact 3D reconstruction or more accurate rebinning methods [Kinahan and Karp, 1994].

The rebinning of data via SSRB can be achieved on-line with most commercial volume PET scanners. Even though the data compression entails some loss of position information, SSRB may in some cases be the sole practical approach to routine 3D dynamic scanning.

More accurate rebinning algorithms have been developed to overcome the limitations of the SSRB approximation. The first one is *multi-slice rebinning* (MSRB) [Lewitt et al., 1994]. This method is also very fast and can be performed on-line. The accuracy and resolution is comparable to that of the 3DRP method, but the stability with respect to noise is somewhat inferior.

The second method is the Fourier rebinning algorithm (FORE) [Defrise et al., 1997], which has good accuracy and stability properties for axial apertures at least up to 35 degrees [Matej et al., 1998]. FORE is based on taking the 2D Fourier transform of each oblique sinogram with respect to ϕ and x_r:

$$S(\upsilon_{xr},k,z,\Delta r)=\int_{-\infty}^{+\infty}dx_r\int_0^{2\pi}d\phi\, e^{-2\pi i x_r \upsilon_{xr}}s(x_r,\phi,z,\Delta r)$$

Note that the Fourier transform with respect to ϕ is a periodic Fourier transform, and therefore k is an integer index, whereas υ_{xr} is a real (continuous) frequency as in equation 2.15. The FORE algorithm is based on the frequency-distance relationship [Edholm et al., 1986]: this approximate property states that the value of $S(\upsilon_{xr},k,z,\Delta r)$ depends only upon the value of the tracer distribution $f(\mathbf{x})$ at the points located at a distance $t=-k/(2\pi\upsilon_{xr})$ along the LORs. The distance t is measured on the transaxial projection of the LOR, with $t = 0$ corresponding to the mid-point of the LOR. Clearly, knowing the position t along the LOR, and the angle $\theta\approx\arctan(\Delta r/2R)$ of the LOR, one can assign $S(\upsilon_{xr},k,z,\Delta r)$ to a well defined transaxial slice with axial coordinate $z=z+t\tan\theta$.

The main steps of the FORE algorithm are:

(1) initialize a stack of Fourier transform rebinned sinograms $S_{2D}(\upsilon_{xr},k,z)=0$

(2) for each oblique sinogram $(z, \Delta r)$,

(2.1) Take the 2D Fourier transform to get $S(\upsilon_{xr},k,z,\Delta r)$

(2.2) for each frequency (υ_{xr},k) :

- calculate the plane location $z'=z-k\tan\theta/(2\pi\upsilon_{xr})$

- add $S(\upsilon_{xr},k,z,\Delta r)$ to $S_{2D}(\upsilon_{xr},k,z')$

(3) normalize $S_{2D}(\upsilon_{xr},k,z)$ to take into account the variable number of times each frequency component has been incremented

(4) take the inverse 2D Fourier transform to get for each slice z the rebinned sinogram, $s_{2D}(x_r,\phi,z)$.

The actual implementation is slightly more complex, mainly because a different strategy is used to handle the low values of the υ_{xr} frequencies, [Defrise et al., 1997]. The FORE procedure is an order of magnitude faster than the 3DRP algorithm, but, in contrast with the SSRB and MSRB algorithms, FORE rebinning cannot be performed on-line during data acquisition. Therefore, FORE requires the acquisition of full 3D data sets.

ITERATIVE TECHNIQUES.

Iterative reconstruction techniques for 2D imaging were described earlier. Apart from the system model, which is related to the geometry of data acquisition, iterative algorithms are conceptually independent of the 2- or 3-dimensional nature of the problem, and all techniques developed for 2D PET can in principle be applied to 3D data. The choice of an algorithm and its performance is nevertheless influenced by the properties of the 3D problem. The main property is the data size: the number of equations (LORs) usually exceeds 10 million and, even though the total number of voxels is the same as in 2D, no factorization in slices is possible and hence all voxels must be processed simultaneously.

The need to store such a large transition matrix is a major difficulty when implementing iterative methods. With sufficiently simple models of the measurement, it is possible to take advantage of the sparseness and of the symmetries of the system matrix **A**, but even so the required storage is large (of the order of 0.5 Gbytes for a brain size object [Johnson et al., 1995]). A very simple model may also allow the on-line calculation of the matrix elements. It might be thought that the larger dimension of the problem should result in unacceptably long reconstruction times. Indeed, many methods such as the EM-ML algorithm involve at each iteration one backprojection and one re-projection of the whole data set, and each iteration takes roughly the same time as a full 3D FBP reconstruction. Preliminary studies, however, suggest that fewer iterations are required in 3D to achieve an equivalent accuracy to 2D studies, owing probably to the redundancy of the 3D data [Matej et al., 1994]. Furthermore, the use of fast iterative algorithms such as OSEM [Hudson and Larkin, 1994; Johnson et al., 1995], and the use of smooth basis functions instead of voxels may also accelerate convergence [Furuie et al., 1994]. For example, a 3D implementation of the Algebraic Reconstruction Technique (ART) algorithm with smooth basis functions was observed to accurately reconstruct 3D data in essentially one iteration (that is, one pass through the whole data set), with a reconstruction time similar to that with 3DRP [Matej et al., 1994]. Finally, another promising approach consists of applying a 2D iterative reconstruction method to data rebinned using one of the rebinning methods described above. An example of this approach is combining FORE rebinning with 2D-OSEM [Kinahan et al., 1996].

In conclusion, the iterative reconstruction of large 3D data sets does not seem impractical, even though considerable work remains to be done to develop and rigorously evaluate clinically useful algorithms. The benefits to be expected from iterative algorithms are (1) improved resolution from a more accurate modeling of the physical measurement [Liow et al., 1997; Qi et al., 1998], and (2) a decreased variance in the reconstructed image, especially in low uptake regions [Kinahan et al., 1996].

Noise

Image quality in PET is often limited by statistical noise. Increasing sensitivity is therefore an important goal when designing new scanners, and in this respect the introduction of 3D acquisition has been an important step in the development of PET. The increased sensitivity achieved by 3D acquisition, however, is useful only insofar as it leads to improved image quality. This entails two conditions. The first one is that the systematic error (the *bias*) should not be degraded significantly by the increased scatter and random background. This problem is discussed in chapter 3. The second condition is that the *variance* in the reconstructed image is actually improved by the increased sensitivity. This problem is briefly discussed in this section. As a rigorous analysis of the 3DRP algorithm in the presence of noise is impractical, we first consider a simple model with a set of complete 2D projections reconstructed using the 3D FBP method. Next the 3DRP algorithm and the consequences of the spatial non-uniformity of the sensitivity are discussed.

NOISE PROPAGATION BY THE 3D FBP ALGORITHM.

The variance in an image reconstructed using 3D FBP can be easily calculated if one assumes a set of complete 2D projections (with $0 \le \phi < \pi$ and $|\theta| \le \Theta_c$) with the number of coincidences detected in each LOR distributed as an independent Poisson variable. Consider for instance a uniformly labeled, non-attenuating, sphere of diameter d and denote by N the total number of detected coincidences. The variance of a voxel at the center of the sphere is then approximately equal to [Defrise et al., 1990]:

$$\text{variance} \approx \frac{1}{N}\left(\frac{d}{2l}\right)^4 k(\Theta) = \frac{3}{4\pi n_V}\left(\frac{d}{2l}\right)k(\Theta) \tag{2.42}$$

where l is the voxel size (assumed isotropic), k is a function of the scanner's aperture and of the reconstruction filter used, and n_V is the number of events per voxel. Although equation 2.42 is derived from a simplified model, it leads to two important conclusions:

(1) For a fixed filter (for example Colsher's filter with a Hamming window) the value of k is found to be almost constant when Θ varies from 0 (corresponding to the limit of a 2D acquisition with slice by slice reconstruction) to 20 degrees (for a 3D acquisition with a typical volume scanner). Hence the noise behavior of the 3D and 2D FBP are similar, and this can be explained by the fact that both the ramp filter and Colsher's filter are proportional to the modulus of the frequency. A consequence is that the gain in sensitivity, that is, the larger value of N in a 3D acquisition, is fully translated into an improvement of the image variance.

(2) Another remarkable property of equation 2.42 is the dependence on the voxel size. When l is divided by 2, e.g. to reflect the improvement of the detector resolution, the number of counts N must be multiplied by 16 if the reconstructed variance is to be kept constant. Though this rule should not be taken strictly, it suggests that full benefit cannot be taken of an improvement of the detector resolution unless it is accompanied by a significant increase of the sensitivity. This is why under-sampling techniques such as mashing (which are roughly equivalent to increasing l) are often used for low count studies with modern high resolution PET scanners.

In the presence of scatter and random background, the data are no longer distributed as Poisson variables. Equation 2.42 nevertheless remains approximately valid if one replaces the number of counts N by the number of noise equivalent counts (N_{NEC}), which is defined in chapter 3. Note that the variance calculated in this way does not account for any bias not removed by the scatter and random corrections.

Equation 2.42 is given for a voxel at the center of a uniform sphere, in the absence of attenuation. A more detailed study of the variance can be found in [Defrise et al., 1990]. In general, the variance in an image reconstructed using 3D FBP is dominated by the attenuation correction and varies only smoothly, even when the tracer is not uniformly distributed. With an iterative algorithms such as the ML-EM algorithm, in contrast, the variance is an increasing function of the local value tracer uptake $f(x,y,z)$ [Barrett et al., 1994], and in low activity regions lower variance can be obtained with these algorithms than with FBP.

NON STATIONARITY OF THE RECONSTRUCTED VARIANCE.

The previous analysis assumed complete 2D projections containing non-correlated Poisson noise. This hypothesis does not hold with the 3DRP algorithm, because the synthetic projection data estimated from the 2D image are not distributed as independent Poisson variables. Furthermore, the relative contribution of the synthetic data depends on the position within the field-of-view. This contribution is minimum at $z = 0$ and maximum for the end planes at $z = \pm L_D/2$. The noise behavior of the 3DRP algorithm is therefore complex to analyze. However, the dependence of the reconstructed image variance upon the position within the field-of-view is chiefly governed by two factors:

(1) the *local sensitivity* $\varepsilon(x,y,z)$, is proportional to the solid angle subtended by the scanner at a point (x,y,z). The number of events per voxel in equation 2.42, n_V, will now be proportional to $\varepsilon(x,y,z)$. This function is almost constant in each transverse plane as long as the radius of the transaxial FOV is small compared to the scanner radius R_D. The axial sensitivity profile is approximately trapezoidal, and given by:

$$\varepsilon(0,0,z) = \begin{cases} cR_D \sin(\Theta), & 0 < |z| < \dfrac{L_D}{2} - z_o \\ cL_D/2 - |z|, & \dfrac{L_D}{2} - z_o < |z| < \dfrac{L_D}{2} \end{cases}$$

where c is a constant, Θ is the maximum value of θ incorporated in the reconstruction (fig. 2.6), and $z_o = R_D \tan(\Theta)$. An example is shown in fig. 2.25 for Θ equal to the scanner aperture Θ_D, (solid line) and for $\Theta = 0.75\Theta_D$ (dashed line).

In the case of $\Theta = 0.75\Theta_D$, the amount of data to estimate and to backproject is significantly reduced as compared to $\Theta = \Theta_D$, while the total loss of sensitivity, due to discarding data with the largest $|\theta|$ values does not exceed about 25%, as can be seen by comparing the areas under the two profiles in fig. 2.25. A practical implication of the axial non-uniformity of the variance is that the axial interval between successive bed positions in a 3D whole body study must be smaller than the length of the scanner to maintain a uniform sensitivity [Cutler and Xu, 1995; Badawi et al., 1997].

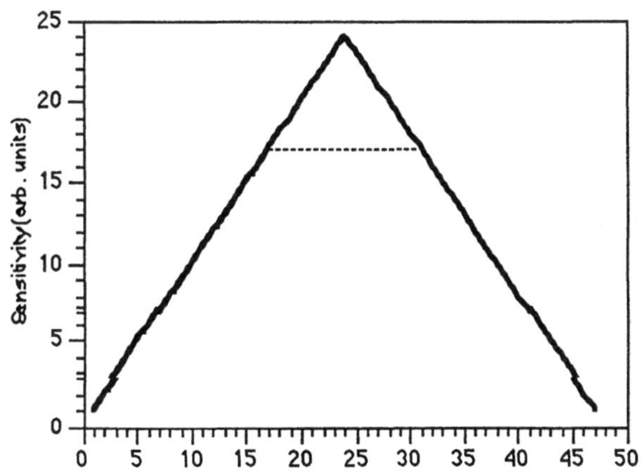

Figure 2.25 Sensitivity profile for a 3D PET scanner as a function of axial position for two different values of the maximum projection angles incorporated into the reconstruction.

(2) the second factor influencing image variance is the *smoothing effect* of the 3DRP algorithm. The truncated data are obtained by forward projecting the initial image estimate reconstructed from the 2D data subset, and this complex reconstruction-reprojection procedure generates estimated data having lower variance than the measured data. After applying 3D FBP, the image variance will therefore be decreased in the high $|z|$ regions where a significant fraction of the data have been estimated rather than measured. This variance reduction depends on the types of interpolation and apodization used in the 2D reconstruction and in the reprojection step.

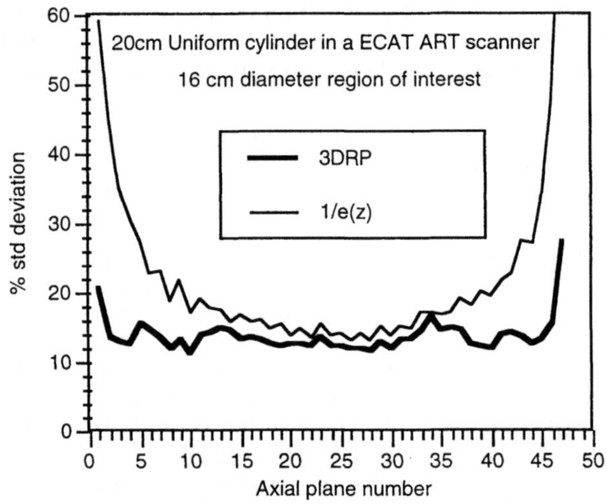

Figure 2.26 Variance in a transverse image slice versus axial position of slice.

As an example, fig. 2.26 shows the reconstructed variance in each slice of a uniform cylinder reconstructed from 3D data. The reciprocal of the sensitivity, $1/\varepsilon(z)$ is also shown, demonstrating the difference in variance reduction for the external slices due to the 3DRP reprojection step.

Note that the reduced variance for 3DRP, which partly compensates the drop of sensitivity near the edges of the scanner, is specific to the 3DRP algorithm and is not observed with other 3D methods (Favor, Direct Fourier Reconstruction) or rebinning methods SSRB, MSRB, and FORE. For these algorithms, the variance closely follows the $1/\varepsilon(z)$ profile. The tradeoff in the 3DRP algorithm for the reduction in variance at the axial ends of the FOV is a slight loss in resolution [Defrise et al., 1994; Kinahan and Karp, 1994].

References

Badawi RD, Marsden PK, Cronin BF, Sutcliffe JL, Maisey MN. Optimization of noise-equivalent count rates in 3D PET. Phys Med Biol 1997;41:1755-1776.

Barrett HH, Swindell W. Radiological Imaging. New York: Academic Press, 1981.

Barrett HH, Wilson DW, Tsui BMW. Noise properties of the EM algorithm: I. Theory. Phys Med Biol 1994;39:833-846.

Cheung WK, Lewitt RM. Modified Fourier reconstruction method using shifted transform samples. Phys Med Biol 1991;36:269-277.

Colsher JG. Fully three-dimensional positron emission tomography. Phys Med Biol 1980;25:103-115.

Cutler PD, Xu M. Strategies to improve 3D whole body PET image reconstruction. J Nuc Med 1995;36:93-94.

Daube-Witherspoon ME, Muehllehner G. Treatment of axial data in three-dimensional PET. J Nuc Med 1987;28:1717-1724.

Deans SR. The Radon transform and some of its applications. New York: Wiley, 1983.

Defrise M, Geissbuhler A, Townsend DW. Performance study of 3D reconstruction algorithms for PET. Phys Med Biol 1994;39.

Defrise M, Kinahan PE, Townsend DW, Michel C, Sibomana M, Newport D. Exact and approximate rebinning algorithms for 3D PET data. IEEE Trans Med Imag 1997;16:145-158.

Defrise M, Townsend DW, Clack R. FaVoR: A fast reconstruction algorithm for volume imaging in PET. Proceedings of the IEEE Nuclear Science Symposium and Medical Imaging Conference; 1991 November 2-9; Santa Fe, NM;1919-1923.

Defrise M, Townsend DW, Deconinck F. Statistical noise in three-dimensional positron tomography. Phys Med Biol 1990;35:131-138.

Edholm PR, Lewitt RM, Lindholm B. Novel Properties of the Fourier Decomposition of the Sinogram. Proceedings of the International Workshop on Physics and Engineering of Computerized Multidimensional Imaging and Processing; 1986; Proceedings of the SPIE 671:8-18.

Egger M. Fast Volume reconstruction in positron emission tomography. [PhD Thesis]. Laussane, University of Laussane, 1996.

Fessler JA. Penalized weighted least squares image reconstruction for positron emission tomography. IEEE Trans Med Imag 1994;13(2):290-300.

Furuie SS, Herman GT, Narayan TK, Kinahan PE, Karp JS, Lewitt RM, Matej S. A methodology for testing for statistically significant differences between fully 3D PET reconstruction algorithms. Phys Med Biol 1994;39:341-354.

Herbert T, Leahy RM. A generalized EM algorithm for 3-D Bayesian reconstruction for Poisson data using Gibbs priors. IEEE Trans Med Imag 1989;MI-8:194-202.

Hudson H, Larkin R. Accelerated image reconstruction using ordered subsets of projection data. IEEE Trans Med Imag 1994;13:601-609.

Jackson JI, Meyer CH, Nishimura DG, Macovski A. Selection of a convolution function for Fourier inversion using gridding. IEEE Trans Med Imag 1991;10:473-478.

Johnson CA, Yan Y, Carson RE, Martino RL, Daube-Witherspoon ME. A system for the 3D reconstruction of retracted-septa data using the EM algorithm. IEEE Trans Nuc Sci 1995;42:1223-1227.

Kak AC, Slaney M. Principles of Computerized Tomographic Imaging. New York: IEEE Press, 1988.

Kinahan PE, Karp JS. Figures of Merit for comparing reconstruction algorithms with a volume-imaging PET scanner. Phys Med Biol 1994;39:631-638.

Kinahan PE, Michel C, Defrise M, Townsend DW, Sibomana M, Lonneux M, Newport DF, Luketich JD. Fast Iterative Image Reconstruction of 3D PET Data. Proceedings of the IEEE Nuclear Science Symposium and Medical Imaging Conference; 1996 November 5-8; Anaheim, CA;1918-1922.

Kinahan PE, Rogers JG. Analytic 3D image reconstruction using all detected events. IEEE Trans Nuc Sci 1989;36:964-968.

Lewitt RM, Muehllehner G, Karp JS. Three-dimensional image reconstruction for PET by multi-slice rebinning and axial image filtering. Phys Med Biol 1994;39:321-339.

Liow J-S, Strother SC, Rehm K, Rottenburg A. Improved resolution for PET volume-imaging through three-dimensional iterative reconstruction. J Nuc Med 1997;38:1623-1630.

Matej S, Herman GT, Narayan TK, Furuie SS, Lewitt RM, Kinahan PE. Evaluation of task-oriented performance of several fully 3-D PET reconstruction algorithms. Phys Med Biol 1994;39:355-367.

Matej S, Karp JS, Lewitt RM, Becher AJ. Performance of the Fourier Rebinning Algorithm for PET with Large Acceptance Angles. Phys Med Biol 1998;43.

Natterer F. The Mathematics of Computerized Tomography. New York: Wiley, 1986.

Orlov SS. Theory of three-dimensional image reconstruction: I Conditions for a complete set of projections. Soviet Physics Crystallography 1976;20:429-433.

Orlov SS. Theory of three-dimensional image reconstruction: II The recovery operator. Soviet Physics Crystallography 1976;20:429-433.

Qi J, Leahy RM, Cherry SR, Chatziioannou A, Farquhar TH. High Resolution 3D Bayesian Image Reconstruction Using the Small Animal microPET Scanner. Phys Med Biol 1998;43.

Shepp LA, Vardi Y. Maximum likelihood reconstruction for emission tomography. IEEE Trans Med Imag 1982;2:113-119.

Sossi V, Stazyk M, Kinahan PE, Ruth T. Implementation of a 3D acquisition and 2D reconstruction technique on an ECAT 953B for phantom and human basal ganglia studies. J Comp Assist Tomogr 1994;18:1004-1010.

Stearns CW, Chesler DA, Brownell GL. Accelerated image reconstruction for a cylindrical positron tomograph using Fourier domain methods. IEEE Trans Nuc Sci 1990;37:773-777.

Stearns CW, Crawford CR, Hu H. Oversampled filters for quantitative volumetric PET reconstruction. Phys Med Biol 1994;39:381-388.

Townsend DW, Defrise M. Image reconstruction methods in positron tomography. CERN;Technical Report. 1993.

Chapter 3. QUANTITATIVE PROCEDURES IN 3D PET

Dale L. Bailey

MRC Cyclotron Unit, Hammersmith Hospital
London, UK

with contributions from:

Maria-Carla Gilardi, Sylke Grootoonk, Paul Kinahan, Claude Nahmias, John Ollinger, David Townsend , Regine Trébossen, and Margharita Zito

Introduction

Positron tomography has always had a strong quantitative emphasis. The reconstructed volumes which result from 2D acquisition provide radioactivity concentrations accurate to within a few percent under well-controlled, calibrated conditions. This is mostly due to the low acceptance of scattered coincidences and the accuracy of the corrections for random coincidences, dead time, and attenuation. In 3D PET though, many of these factors are altered by the acquisition geometry and the procedures needed for 3D reconstruction. This chapter discusses the approaches taken at present to applying the various corrections needed for quantitative 3D PET.

STEPS IN RECONSTRUCTING DATA FROM 3D PET

As an introduction, fig. 3.1 shows schematically the data required and the processing steps needed to perform a quantitative reconstruction in 3D PET. The procedure depicted uses the reprojection algorithm [Kinahan and Rogers, 1989; Townsend et al., 1989], although, as seen in Chapter 2, it is only one of a number of approaches available. The reprojection algorithm is the most common method in use at the time of writing. In general, four sets of data are required to produce a quantitative 3D reconstruction: (i) the emission data to be reconstructed; accurate correction for attenuation requires (ii) a transmission and, (iii), a corresponding blank scan, and finally (iv) correction factors to normalize the emission data for differences in detector efficiencies and geometric effects. Each aspect of this procedure will be examined in the following sections, starting with a number of approaches to correcting for scattered photons. Note that random coincidences are currently subtracted in 3D PET in the

B. Bendriem and D.W. Townsend (eds.) The Theory and Practice of 3D PET, 55-109.

same way as they are in 2D PET.

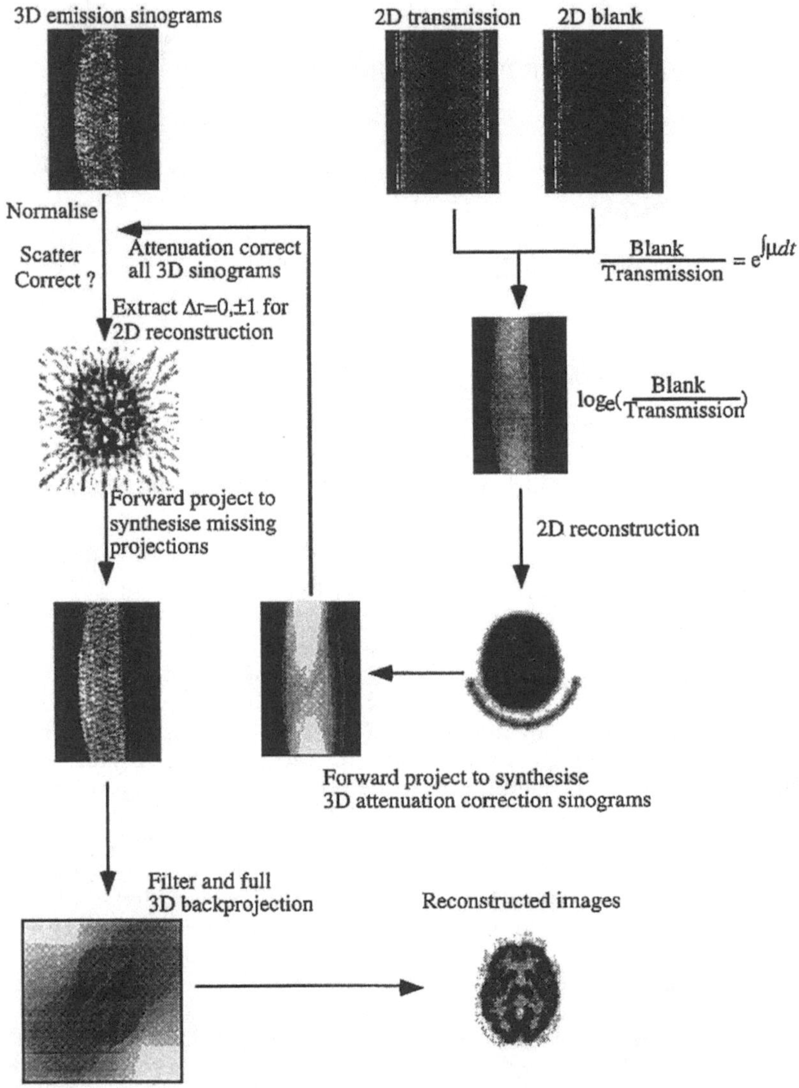

Figure 3.1. The steps in reconstructing data acquired in 3D PET using the reprojection algorithm are shown.

Scatter in 3D PET Measurements

The most significant distinction affecting quantification in 3D PET compared with 2D PET is the greater acceptance of scattered coincidences. Scatter *qualitatively* decreases contrast by misplacing events during reconstruction, and *quantitatively* causes errors in the reconstructed radioactivity concentrations. Scatter is increased by two to threefold in 3D PET compared with 2D, and may constitute 50% or more of the total recorded events. In 2D PET the fraction of events scattered is typically less than 15% of the total acquired events. In addition, the presence of some scatter in the transmission data helps to quantitatively "offset" the scatter in the emission data by underestimating the attenuation correction factors in much the same way that an "effective μ value" has been used in SPECT [Larsson, 1980]. Scatter fraction, which is defined as the ratio of scattered to total (*i.e.*, scattered plus unscattered) events, is affected by the energy window selected, the scintillation crystal, the dimensions of the detectors, the tomograph length and diameter, and the size and density of the object.

In positron emission tomography, photons resulting from the positron-electron annihilation can interact with the surrounding atoms as they propagate from their origin. Interactions of photons with an energy of 0.511 MeV are almost totally via the Compton effect, an elastic scattering after collision with a weakly bound orbital electron [Compton, 1923]. The results of this interaction are ionisation of the atom and change of direction and energy of the photon. The loss in energy is used to overcome the weak binding energy of the electron and contribute kinetic energy to the ejected Compton electron. The energy of the photon after the Compton interaction (E_γ') is given by:

$$E_\gamma' = \frac{E_\gamma}{1+\frac{E_\gamma}{m_0c^2}(1-\cos[\theta_c])} \qquad [3.1]$$

where E_γ is the incident photon energy (in MeV), m_0c^2 is the rest-mass equivalent energy of the electron, and θ_c is the scattering angle of the photon. Due to the limited energy resolution of the scintillation detectors used in PET scanners - typically 10%-30% FWHM at 0.511 MeV - rejection of scattered photons on the basis of energy discrimination is limited. In general, scattered photons decrease overall image contrast as their lines-of-response are incorrect and will be attributed to lines of response spatially uncorrelated with their point of origin. This is in contrast to single photon tomographic modalities (SPECT, X-Ray CT), where the scattered photon's apparent line-of-response is collinear with the point at which the scattering took place (fig. 3.2a).

As PET utilises coincidence counting for electronic collimation, the effect on the line-of-response of the event after scattering is not as straightforward. The line-of-response assigned is one which joins the pair of detectors which recorded the photons and can appear quite unrelated to the photon's origin, as can be seen in fig. 3.2b. In single photon tomography scattering appears only within the object, whereas in PET scatter can appear well outside of the object. Though fig. 3.2 shows a transaxial view of the scattering phenomenon, in the open geometry of 3D PET the same is true in the axial (*z*) dimension as well. As a consequence of the increased acceptance of scatter, the ability to quantify reconstructed radioactivity concentrations in the object is compromised and this is one of the reasons to some extent that fully 3D acquisition and reconstruction in PET was not pursued earlier.

MEASURING SCATTER

Before discussing techniques to correct for scatter it is necessary to characterize the nature of the scatter in 3D PET data. The contribution of scatter can be separated into two global parameters: the *amount* of scatter present in the data, often referred to as the *scatter fraction* and denoted by the symbol k, and the *distribution* of the scattered photons relative to the unscattered data, referred to as the *scatter function*, denoted by κ. The scatter fraction is defined as the ratio of the scattered photons to the total number of photons (including scatter) recorded; a similar term, the *scatter ratio*, is usually taken to be the ratio of the scattered to unscattered events. The scatter fraction will be influenced by various parameters such as the density and thickness of the scintillation detectors, the acceptance angle of the tomograph, and the energy resolution of the detectors and discriminator windows that are used, but will be dominated by the size and density of the object containing the radioactivity. The measurement of scatter fraction has been defined by the Society of Nuclear Medicine and the US National Electrical Manufacturers' Association (SNM/NEMA) for positron tomographs to provide a class standard to allow comparisons between devices [Karp et al., 1991]. Scatter function is a less frequently measured parameter as it is more closely linked with the convolution/ deconvolution and "scatter fitting" approaches to scatter correction. The simplest method that has been used to characterize scatter is to measure a needle source containing a positron emitting radionuclide placed in a uniformly attenuating medium. This approximates a Dirac delta function and allows direct measurement of the system line spread function and scatter profile. The test object suggested by SNM/NEMA is a water-filled cylinder which is 20 cm in diameter.

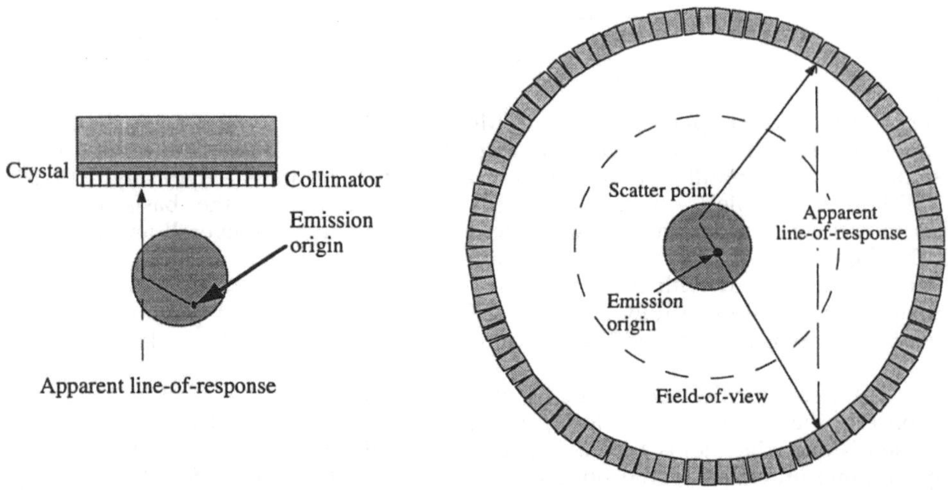

Figure 3.2. Diagram (a) on the left indicates how scatter in SPECT is constrained to appear within the boundaries of the object as only one photon is required for an event to register while in PET, on the right (b), the action of joining the two crystals which detected the photons in coincidence can form a line of response far outside the object.

Fig. 3.3 shows transverse profiles (in s) in the projection space for a ^{68}Ge needle source in (a) a 20 cm diameter water-filled cylinder in 2D, (b) the same in 3D, and, (c) in air. In each case the cylinder is centred on the origin of the graph. It is clear that the boundary (at -10 cm, +10 cm) of the object has no influence on the profile. The profile from the 3D measurement, in particular, demonstrates how well defined the scatter portion of the curve is outside the object, and this has been the impetus to developing the scatter correction methods based on fitting analytical functions to the recorded emission data *outside* the object being studied. For the SNM/NEMA measurement of scatter fraction, data are acquired with the source at three different radial locations. At each location the counts under the total curve and the counts under the estimated scatter portion of the curve (the shaded section of fig. 3.4) are determined and the average scatter fraction calculated from an area weighted average. The scatter function may be found by fitting an appropriate function (*e.g.*, exponential, Gaussian) to the region outside the central peak. One cautionary note should be made regarding the SNM/NEMA evaluation of scatter: it only evaluates scatter in a region to within ±2 cm of the outside of the cylinder.

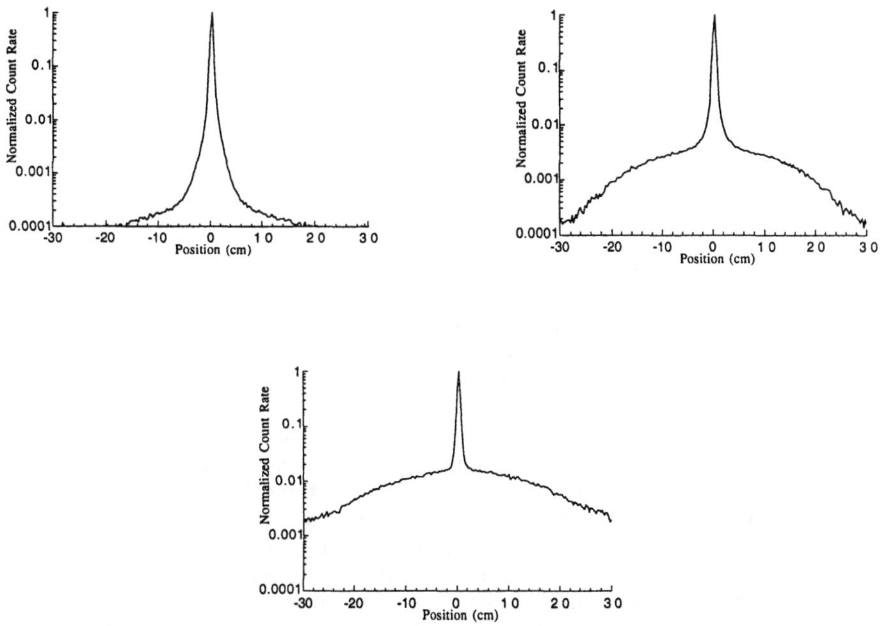

Figure 3.3. Line source profiles of a transaxially centred line source of ^{68}Ge for 2D PET in a 20 cm cylinder (top left), 3D PET in air (top right), and 3D PET in a 20 cm cylinder (bottom).

When using a correction which subtracts scatter estimates from sinograms this may not be appropriate as there is scatter well outside of this region. The SNM/NEMA method is intended as a means of classifying performance and facilitating comparisons between scanners, so the use of the SNM/NEMA scatter fraction in a correction scheme should be considered carefully before use.

An alternative method which has been reported [Bailey and Meikle, 1994] employs a paired measurement of a needle source in air, subsequently attenuated artificially by multiplication with a calculated attenuation correction matrix which has a constant attenuation coefficient (μ=0.095 cm^{-1}) to give a 'narrow-beam' attenuated measurement without scatter, and the actual measurement of the needle in the water-filled cylinder, which is attenuated and will also contain scatter. Comparison of the total counts in these two sets of projections should differ only due to scatter and thus the scatter fraction can be estimated. This method makes few assumptions and gives a measure of the total scatter in the projection data. The scatter fraction measured in this manner was used in their implementation of the convolution-subtraction correction method. While the transaxial profiles demonstrate the increase in scatter in 3D (see fig. 3.3) within a plane, the positron annihilations contributing to the measurement arise predominantly outside of the plane being considered.

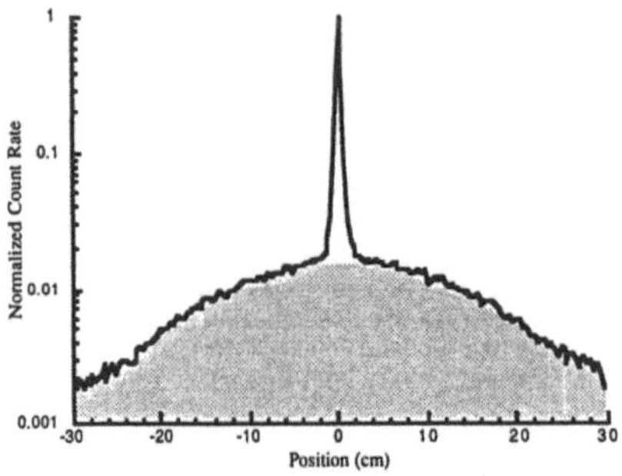

Figure 3.4. The portion under the shaded section is regarded as scatter in most approaches. In the SNM/NEMA measurement the scatter is restricted to -12 cm - +12 cm (2 cm beyond the cylinder) on this graph for a 20 cm diameter cylinder.

This is because it is the removal of septa and increase in acceptance angle which increases the scatter recorded. We assume that the scatter arising from within a particular plane is the same for 2D and 3D PET, as there is no collimation in plane using septa in 2D PET. The major difference in scatter acceptance between 2D and 3D PET is due to axial scattering from outside of the plane being considered. The scatter characterization method of Cherry [Cherry et al., 1993] measures this out of plane component directly by examining the differences between 2D and 3D acquisitions of the same object. The method is impractical with radionuclide distributions which are changing rapidly, though. Fig. 3.5 shows the axial profile of scatter for a line source oriented in the x-y plane of the tomograph, as indicated in the figure at the top of the graph. The scatter in 2D is seen to be almost identical in air or in a scattering medium, while in 3D there is increased axial scattering. Interestingly, there appears to be an extended "tail" in the 3D air measurement as well. It might have been anticipated that this measurement should overlay the 2D air measurement, but it clearly extends further with a reasonably constant value. This appears slightly exaggerated in the graph as the entire field of view is only 10.8 cm for this tomograph (ECAT 953B), so that the length of the low level "background" is only ±3 cm or so. However, it is an unexpected finding which is possibly due to scatter off the gantry itself, and emphasises how the open geometry of 3D PET allows for greatly increased scatter acceptance.

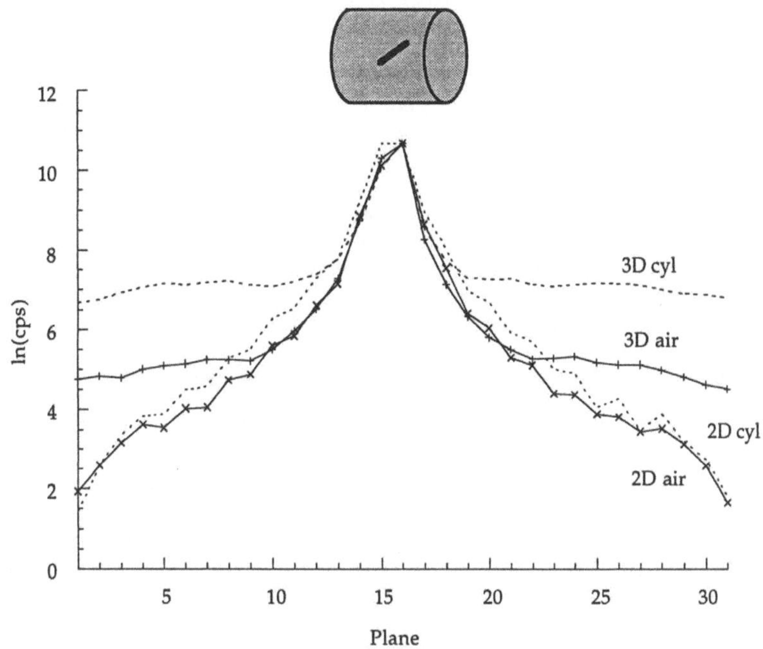

Figure 3.5. Axial scatter in 2D and 3D (see text for further discussion).

Assessing the Accuracy of Scatter Correction

Scatter correction methods differ from each other in the assumptions and methods adopted to model the scatter component within the photopeak energy window. As scatter events cannot be experimentally distinguished from true photopeak events, simulation techniques are often employed to "estimate" the scatter component. In assessing the accuracy of scatter correction the overriding goal must be accurate *absolute* quantification. Reports of the performance of scatter correction algorithms which quote "relative concentrations" must, we feel, be viewed with cautious optimism until careful calibration confirms that the measurements are accurate in units of radioactive decay per unit volume.

The following approaches have been adopted to assessing the accuracy of scatter correction methods.

SCATTER CORRECTION OF MONTE CARLO SIMULATED 3D DATA

The true scatter component (being an experimentally impossible measurement) can be obtained only by simulations. For this purpose Monte Carlo techniques can be used, simulating the physics of the PET detection process. Given a known radioactive source distribution and density of the object, Monte Carlo techniques allow detected events to be classified into non-scattered and scattered events and the scatter component to be determined in an independent way. However, the following considerations in the use of Monte Carlo simulations have to be borne in mind:

- Monte Carlo techniques can produce a "true" scatter component only for situations where the source geometry is known. This can be tested with simulated phantom studies, but does not lend itself readily to clinical studies, however;

- Monte Carlo simulations are time consuming and it is hard to generate statistically significant data. In symmetrical objects, with identical projections, a single projection averaged over all angles can be generated, improving signal/noise ratio. However simulating symmetrical objects further reduces the generality of the approach;

- Monte Carlo simulations themselves must be experimentally validated.

ASSESSING SCATTER CORRECTION BY EXPERIMENTAL METHODS

Testing with Phantoms. The use of experimental phantom data is the most universally applied approach for assessing the accuracy of scatter correction methods. In phantoms, the distribution is known (in terms of both the density of the object and the spatial distribution of the radioactivity) and the radioactivity concentration in the various compartments can be accurately measured by sampling aliquots that can be counted in a calibrated secondary detector. This approach measures absolute quantification. A major consideration in using phantoms, however, is that phantoms are limited to situations generally described by simple geometrical structures (*e.g.*, line sources, spheres, cylinders, *etc.*) and this might limit the generality of the approach. However, more complicated phantoms currently exist (*e.g.*, Hoffman 3D Brain phantom, *etc.*), which attempt to emulate clinical conditions in a realistic way. One test object designed with the aim of testing scatter correction specifically is the so-called "Utah phantom" (devised at the *2nd International Meeting on Fully Three-Dimensional Image Reconstruction in Radiology and Nuclear Medicine,* held in Snowbird, Utah in 1993, hence the name [Townsend et al., 1994b]). The Utah phantom is a 20 cm diameter cylinder containing various compartments. An X-Ray CT scan of the phantom is shown in fig. 3.6.

Examples of the Utah phantom demonstrating various relative concentrations in the different compartments for a single slice are shown in fig. 3.7, from a series of 4 different experiments. The phantom allows independent access to each of the compartments and some typical uses for each of the compartments include:

- compartment A: a uniform radioactivity concentration region; also provides a compartment to test scattering from outside of the coincidence event field of view;

- compartment B: the general "background" region, with or without radioactivity;

- compartment C: provides an annular region giving a distribution roughly approximating a cortical grey matter pattern;

- compartments D and E: may be filled with radioactivity concentration greater or less than the surrounding region B; may contain different density material.

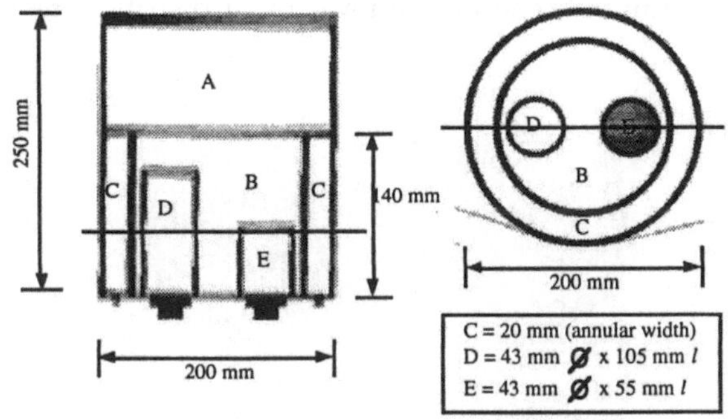

Figure 3.6. Axial (left) and transverse (right) X-Ray CT sections through the Utah phantom with dimensions are shown. The position of the thin horizontal lines indicate the level of the section on the alternate image. For the CT scan the phantom was emptied so that the phantom contained perspex and air only.

Reports of the effect of scatter correction on the Utah phantom have started to appear [Townsend et al., 1996; Watson et al., 1996]. The convolution-subtraction scatter correction method was applied to this object in 3D for a variety of radioactivity concentrations in the compartments, with uniform density (water) in all compartments and with all the radioactivity essentially within the field of view.

Measurements with compartments filled with low density material (sawdust) demonstrated a tendency of the technique to overestimate the amount of scatter present. This manifests itself, as we saw previously, in clinical studies as well. The Utah phantom may well become a *de facto* standard for testing scatter correction.

Comparing 2D and 3D PET Scans to Assess Scatter Correction. Cherry proposed a method for scatter correction in which both 2D and 3D PET data of the object are acquired and the difference determined [Cherry et al., 1993]. 2D PET data, properly corrected for scatter and attenuation can be assumed to provide a quantitatively accurate estimate of radioactivity distribution in the source object. The radioactivity distribution can be compared in 3D and 2D, with the 2D scan representing a (scatter-free) reference. The major limitation of this approach as a scatter correction method is that it requires a separate scan to be performed in 2D, and this is not always possible as the radionuclide distribution can change rapidly, especially for dynamic studies. However, as pointed out by Cherry, this method does provide an excellent approach for assessing other scatter correction methods.

The accuracy of scatter correction should be assessed in terms of the capability to recover radioactivity concentration ratios in both "cold" and "hot" regions of radioactivity. Likewise, the accuracy in phantoms of heterogeneous density must also be addressed; studies to date have tended to concentrate on cerebral applications. An ideal scatter correction should be effective in the case of distributed sources (as in brain perfusion studies) and in the case of activity concentrated in isolated regions (as in receptors or monoclonal antibody tumour studies). In particular, not only symmetrical but also asymmetrical source distributions should be considered. Noise effects have not been discussed explicitly here, but the accuracy of the correction needs to be validated over a wide dynamic range of total counts in the data. This will be extremely important for methods which use multiple energy windows, or fit distributions to data outside of the object.

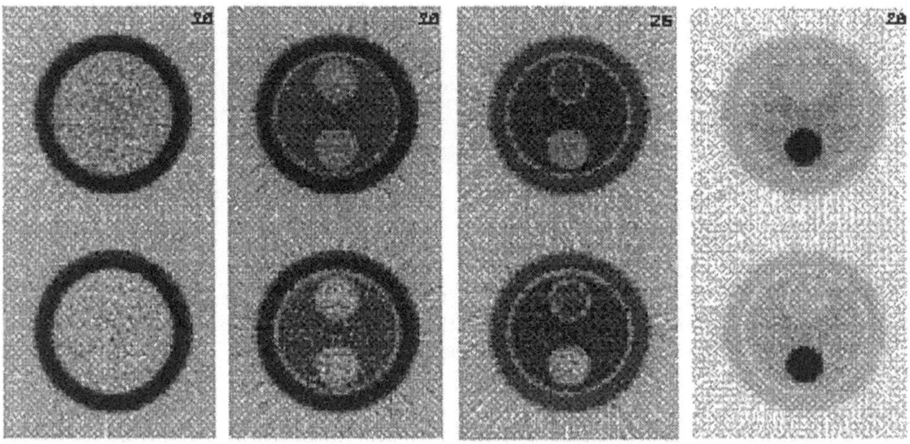

Figure 3.7. The Utah phantom is shown for four different experiments with different relative concentrations of radioactivity in the compartments. All studies were acquired in 3D on the ECAT 953B at Hammersmith Hospital. The top row shows the data without scatter correction, while the bottom row shows the reconstructed images after the convolution-subtraction scatter correction. In the pair of images on the left, compartment C only contains radioactivity, while compartments B, D, and E contain water. In the next pair of images, radioactivity has been added to compartment B. In the 3rd pair of images radioactivity of concentration lower than that of compartment B has been added to compartment D, while in the final images a radioactivity concentration 10 times that of compartment B has been added to compartment E. The inaccuracies in the absolute concentrations reconstructed in the uncorrected data (top row) ranged between +13% - +49% in these experiments (+3% - +12% in 2D without scatter correction), while after correction these errors were reduced to -9% - +3% (-12% - +3% in 2D with scatter correction).

Scatter Correction

OVERVIEW OF CURRENT APPROACHES

A number of approaches to scatter correction in emission tomography in general have been proposed and these fall into three broad categories [Bailey et al., 1994]:

- Energy window manipulations
    - asymmetric window about the photopeak [Koral et al., 1986],
    - dual windows over photopeak and a lower ("scatter") window in SPECT

[Jaszczak et al., 1984] and 3D PET [Grootoonk et al., 1991; Shao et al., 1993],

- splitting the photopeak with a pair of windows [King et al., 1992; Pretorious et al., 1993; Naude et al., 1996],
- multiple windows [Gagnon et al., 1989; Penney et al., 1991; Bendriem et al., 1993; Bentourkia et al., 1993; Shao et al., 1994; Bentourkia et al., 1995; Haynor et al., 1995],
- on-line correction with energy-weighted acquisition [DeVito et al., 1989],

- Pre- or post-reconstruction filtering and/or subtraction operations such as
  - Metz or Weiner filtering [King et al., 1984; Links et al., 1992],
  - deconvolution [Bergström et al., 1983; Floyd et al., 1985; Townsend et al., 1991; McKee et al., 1992; Prati et al., 1993],
  - convolution-subtraction [Axelsson et al., 1984; Msaki et al., 1987; Bailey et al., 1989a; Yanch et al., 1990; Meikle et al., 1991; Shao and Karp, 1991; Wu et al., 1993; Lercher and Wienhard, 1994],
  - fitting analytical functions (e.g., Gaussian distributions) to the data outside of the object to estimate scatter within the object [Cherry and Huang, 1995; Stearns, 1995],
  - transmission-dependent scatter estimation [Meikle et al., 1991; Meikle et al., 1994],

- Calculating the scatter distribution
  - direct calculation from analytical formulae and source/object geometry [Egbert and May, 1980; Barney et al., 1993; Ollinger and Johns, 1993; Hiltz and McKee, 1994; Ollinger, 1996; Watson et al., 1996],
  - scatter estimation from Monte Carlo calculation [Ljungberg and Strand, 1990; Levin et al., 1995].

A number of the above methods have been implemented for 3D PET and are discussed in the next sections.

ENERGY WINDOW BASED APPROACHES

Multiple energy window methods to correct for scattered photons have been implemented successfully in SPECT for over a decade. In the dual energy window method [Jaszczak et al., 1984], data are simultaneously recorded within a primary photopeak energy window (*e.g.*, 126-154 keV for ^{99m}Tc) and within a secondary lower Compton window (*e.g.*, 95-125 keV). The correction consists of the subtraction of a fraction of the Compton data from the photopeak data. An alternative dual-photopeak window method has also been implemented in SPECT [King et al., 1992; Pretorious et al., 1993] where the photopeak is divided into two energy windows and the scatter fraction in the total photopeak calculated from a regression relation between the counts in the two windows. In the multi-energy window methods [Gagnon et al., 1989] the scattering component within the photopeak window is calculated as a weighted mean of contributions from data recorded within different lower windows.

In PET, the development of the 3D volumetric acquisition mode and improvements in the detector energy resolution have allowed the implementation of scatter corrections based on the analysis of the photon energy. In 3D data acquisition, the contribution of events due to scattered photons is much higher than in 2D (by a factor of 3-5). A large proportion of the scattering contribution in an acquisition plane originates from out-of-plane activity, and out- of-field of view (FOV) activity can also contribute to the scattering. The advantage of energy based approaches is that the effect of the out-of-FOV activity can be monitored by making a measurement in another energy window. Several groups are investigating the potential of acquiring data in two [Grootoonk et al., 1991; Harrison et al., 1991; Bendriem et al., 1993], three [Shao et al., 1994] and multiple energy windows [Bentourkia et al., 1993] to develop corrections for scattering in 3D PET data.

Dual Energy Window Methods. Dual energy window techniques can be classified into two groups: methods estimating the scatter component in the standard acquisition window (including the photopeak) from the events recorded in an energy window placed below the photopeak and methods estimating the unscattered component in the standard window from the unscattered counts recorded in a high energy window in the upper portion of the photopeak. The *dual energy windows* (DEW) technique belongs to the former while the *estimation of trues method* (ETM) belongs to the latter .

Dual Energy Using Photopeak and Scatter Windows. For a standard acquisition energy window of 380-850 keV, the mean scatter fractions for a line source in a 20 cm diameter water-filled cylinder for the ECAT 953B scanner is 0.10 and 0.35 with and without septa respectively [Spinks et al., 1992]. Decreasing the lower level discriminator (LLD) setting from 380 keV to 150 keV increases unscattered counts (by about 20%) as well as increasing scattered events. These are attributed to events which escape from the object unscattered but which either deposit only part of their energy in the detecting crystal, or undergo scatter in the gantry and side-shielding of the scanner. Therefore any energy window selected for this scanner must be assumed to contain both scattered and unscattered events from the object. The counts in the upper (UE) and lower (LE) energy windows in each coincidence line-of-response (LOR) will be given by:

$$UE = UE_{unsc} + UE_{sc} \qquad [3.2a]$$

$$LE = LE_{unsc} + LE_{sc} \qquad [3.2b]$$

where *unsc* and *sc* refer to the unscattered and scattered components respectively. These two equations contain four unknown parameters and so additional data are required to extract the unscattered components. The equations can be re-arranged to give the following expression for scattered counts in the upper window:

$$UE_{sc} = \left[\frac{1}{R_{sc}-R_{unsc}} \cdot LE\right] - \left[\frac{R_{unsc}}{R_{sc}-R_{unsc}} \cdot UE\right] \qquad [3.3]$$

where R_{sc} is the ratio of scattered events (LE_{sc} / UE_{sc}) and R_{unsc} is the ratio of unscattered events (LE_{unsc} / UE_{unsc}) detected. UE_{unsc} can then be obtained from equation (3.2a) by subtracting UE_{sc} from UE.

Practical implementation of the Dual Energy Window Method . In the implementation for an ECAT 953B scanner, coincidence events are assigned to the upper energy window when both photons deposit energy between 380 keV and 850 keV, or to the lower energy window where one or both photons deposit within 200 keV and 380 keV. A 200-380 keV lower window collects approximately one third of the coincidence counts in the upper window. The scaling parameters R_{sc} and R_{unsc} are derived from measurements of the ratios of counts from line sources due to scattered and unscattered events in the two energy windows in a head-sized phantom and in air respectively. R_{unsc} is spatially invariant for a given scanner such that a constant value exists for each sinogram. R_{sc}, however, is found to vary slowly over the transaxial field of view and a single, averaged, value used for each sinogram. Data in each energy window are normalised for detector efficiency and geometry prior to scatter correction. A scaled subtraction of the two energy windows produces an estimate of scatter, UE_{sc}, which is smoothed using a 9 x 9 pixel Gaussian filter prior to subtraction from the upper energy window data to generate the scatter-free sinogram, UE_{unsc}.

In phantoms of uniform attenuation, the dual energy window correction was found to restore the uniformity, contrast and linearity of activity concentration. Relative activity concentrations were restored to within 7% of their true values in the multi-compartment Utah phantom. Importantly, the method was found to provide accurate correction for scattered events arising from activity outside the coincidence field-of-view. In a three-compartment phantom containing water, ^{18}F and ^{11}C, scanned in dynamic, multi-frame mode, the half-lives of the two radionuclides were restored to within ±2% of their true value. The method is applicable to 3-D PET studies of the brain and has been shown to provide unbiased estimates of ligand distribution in comparison with 2D studies in an ECAT 951 whole body scanner [Townsend et al., 1996].

Estimation of Trues Method. In the estimation of trues method, coincidences are acquired simultaneously into two energy windows: a high window with a lower level discriminator higher than 511 keV and a regular acquisition window <u>including</u> the higher window. Both windows have the same UDL value. The rationale for the estimation of trues method is that the number of true unscattered coincidences detected in a given energy range only depends, under stable conditions of temperature and without pile-up effects in the detectors, on the energy settings of the window and the angle of incidence of the photons on the detector face. Thus, the true unscattered counts in the high energy window will simply be related to the true unscattered coincidences in the standard wider window through a function of the energy settings, the radial position in the sinogram for a given line of response and the axial opening angle for a given radial position. This calibrating function is independent of the source distribution. The method is based on results of Monte Carlo simulations demonstrating that only unscattered counts are detected above a critical energy [Thompson, 1993]. Thus, an estimate of the true unscattered counts in the large energy window can be calculated which is subtracted from that acquired in the standard window data to produce a sinogram of scattered coincidences. That sinogram is smoothed and then subtracted from the data recorded in the regular window leading to a scatter-free sinogram. The smoothing step reduces the noise in the newly formed sinogram. Otherwise, noise in the scatter free sinogram would be at least at the same level as in the sinogram acquired in the high energy window.

Practical Implementation of the Estimation of Trues Method. This scatter correction technique has been developed on an ECAT 953B dedicated brain tomograph. The optimal value of the lower level discriminator for the high window was determined from line source measurements. In practice, its choice is a compromise between sensitivity and a residual scatter component. On the ECAT 953B, 625 keV corresponds to the value above which no scattered coincidences are detected in 2D. However, there is a reduction in the sensitivity by a factor of 1000 at that energy threshold. An LLD of 550 keV was used in both the 2D and the 3D modes. Using this value and 650 keV as the high energy setting, the number of true unscattered coincidences is, on average, 1:11 in 2D and 1:9 in 3D to that of the standard window. However, the scattered events represent 6% in 2D and 13% in 3D mainly resulting from small angle Compton scattering. The calibrating function is computed from a line source measurement in air.

The estimation of trues method in 3D provides the same accuracy as the 2D measurement for activity concentration measurements of small spheres inserted in a cold background for diameters greater than 19 mm [Trébossen and Bendriem, 1995a]. Using this method, the quantification of ^{18}F-fluorodopa studies has been demonstrated to be as accurate in 3D as in 2D in normal subjects [Trébossen et al., 1996]. For ^{15}O-water bolus studies, preliminary results obtained in one normal control showed that higher relative differences between activation and rest could be obtained in 3D mode with the estimation of trues correction method, compared with the values measured in the same subject in 2D [Trébossen et al., 1995b].

Comparison of Dual Energy Window Methods Developed in PET. In PET, only unscattered events reach the detector with 511 keV and the number of such coincidences within a given solid angle only depends on the intensity of the radioactive sources. Due to the finite energy resolution of the scintillators, they are detected with a broader energy than 511 keV. In principle, the estimation of trues scatter correction method will be accurate since it attempts to estimate the true unscattered coincidences using a calibrating function of the energy settings independent of the distribution of the radioactive sources. In the dual energy windows method, scattered and unscattered events are recorded in both energy windows. The calibrating function for the scattered coincidences varies with the geometry of the radioactive distribution and the attenuating medium. The measurement of such a function using a 20 cm cylinder is adequate for brain studies. But in the case of non- uniform attenuating medium such as torso studies it may fail to correctly describe the distribution of scattered events. In practice, a small number of scattered coincidences are detected in the high energy window in the estimation of trues technique. However, since they are mostly small angle scatters they could easily be removed using a deconvolution of the scattering response function. One advantage of the dual energy Windows is that a similar number of counts are recorded in both energy windows. This makes it less sensitive to pulse pile-up effects in the detectors than the estimation of trues method. These effects will cause spatial distortions and an over-estimation of the true unscattered events detected in the high energy window in the estimation of trues method. The dual energy windows method may also be less sensitive to temperature variations in the detectors which affects the ratio of events recorded in the two windows in the estimation of trues method. The smoothing process is an important step in both methods. The distribution of scattered counts consists predominantly of low frequency components, thus allowing filtering without degradation of the spatial resolution.

The Triple Energy Window Method. The triple energy window method is an extension of the dual energy window technique. It uses two overlapping windows with the same high energy setting (450 keV), located below the photopeak and a regular window centred on the photopeak and adjacent to the low windows. The ratio of the events recorded in both low energy window for the object and for a uniform cylinder provides a calibrating function that accounts for the distribution of scattered coincidences at low energy. The narrower low energy window is then used with the calibrating function to estimate the scatter component in the regular window.

The Multispectral Acquisition Method. Scatter correction methods based on acquisitions in two or three energy windows make little or no use of the spatial distribution of the scattered events. The spatial distribution of scatter depends on their origin and their contribution varies with the energy. Three components can be distinguished: scattering in the attenuating medium, in the septa and side shielding, and scattering in the detector, characterized by one photon with an energy close to the photopeak and one photon with a lower energy. The multispectral method consists of acquiring data in a very large number (typically 256) windows of the same energy width (16 x 16 energy values for the two photon). In each window, the spatial distribution of each component can be adjusted using mono-exponential functions. The position of the scattered photons in the detectors can be restored thus increasing the sensitivity. Indeed, with this method only 10% of the detected coincidences are rejected. In practice, major drawbacks of such a method include the noise in each window (requiring spatial smoothing) and the number of windows that can be accommodated with the acquisition hardware capabilities of commercial PET systems.

SCATTER CORRECTION BASED ON CONVOLUTION

In the methods based on convolution or deconvolution the distribution of scatter is estimated from the acquired photopeak data. Two parameters are usually required for the scatter estimation and are determined *a priori*: the magnitude of scatter expected (the scatter fraction, k), and the spatial relationship it has with the photopeak data (the scatter function, κ). The imaging model that is used is a purely additive one in which the recorded data are composed of an unscattered and a scattered component [Beck et al., 1969; Erhardt et al., 1974] plus a noise term due to the statistical fluctuations in the data, and which may be written simply as:

$$g_o = g_u + g_s + \eta \qquad [3.4]$$

where g_o are the observed data, g_u and g_s are the unscattered and scattered components respectively, and η is the noise term. As the only measurable quantity (g_o) already contains scatter, the problem is to estimate g_s from g_o, and hence derive the unscattered distribution (g_u).

The convolution-subtraction approach applied in 3D PET **before** reconstruction [Shao et al., 1991; Bailey et al., 1994; Wu et al., 1994] assumes that the convolution of the radionuclide distribution with some scatter function (κ) produces an estimate of the scatter (g_s). Based on the assumption that each point source of emission in the object acts independently, the measured scatter can be related to the unscattered distribution in the object by the convolution relation:

$$\hat{g}_s(x,y) = \int_{-\infty}^{+\infty}\int_{-\infty}^{+\infty} g_u(x',y')\kappa(x-x',y-y')\mathrm{d}x'\mathrm{d}y' \qquad [3.5a]$$

or, using the usual notation and omitting the coordinates:

$$\hat{g}_s = g_u \otimes \kappa \qquad [3.5b]$$

where indicates two-dimensional convolution and the '^' indicates that the parameter is an *estimate* of the scatter. The scatter estimate is then subtracted from g_o after scaling by an appropriate scatter fraction (k). However, as g_u is unknown, the measured g_o is used instead as a first approximation to g_u. As suggested by a number of reports, the process can be repeated iteratively with each step using the previous estimate of the scatter-free distribution as input to the scatter estimation [Bailey et al., 1989b; Shao et al., 1991; Bailey et al., 1994],

$$\hat{g}_u = g_o - k\left(g_o \otimes \kappa\right) \qquad \text{for } n = 1 \qquad [3.6a]$$

$$\hat{g}_u^{(n)} = g_o - k\left(\hat{g}_u^{(n-1)} \otimes \kappa\right) \qquad \text{for } n > 1 \qquad [3.6b]$$

where n is the iteration number. The rationale is that with each iteration the input to the scatter estimation step more closely approximates g_u. A damping factor is sometimes included to prevent oscillation in the result. The novel aspect of this correction method, compared with previous 2D deconvolution approaches, lies in its implementation as a 2D convolution on 2D planar projections (or *planagrams*, with coordinates s,z). This varies from previous convolution/deconvolution methods as these tended to be 1D filtering operations on rows of the sinograms, and therefore did not incorporate out of plane contributions. As this is the biggest difference in scatter between 2D and 3D PET, working with the planagram takes the axial scatter into account. As will be seen later, scatter correction and normalization of the emission data for differences in detector efficiency and geometric effects caused by the circular ring interact strongly. A flow-chart of one implementation of convolution-subtraction scatter correction in 3D PET [Bailey et al., 1994], shown in fig. 3.8, normalises the data before the scatter estimation and correction is performed. In this implementation the scatter estimates are performed using the direct projections only ($\theta \approx 0°$) for tomographs with a limited axial field-of-view, and the output of this convolution is used for all projections which cross the central axis of the scanner at the same point as the direct projection, as the scatter estimates do not vary greatly with slight increases in the polar angle (θ).

Results from Convolution-Subtraction Scatter Correction. The graphs in fig. 3.9 show the effect of this scatter correction on transaxial profiles from attenuation corrected reconstructions of a line source of ^{68}Ge at two different locations: on-axis and displaced by 5 cm radially. The uncorrected data (the upper solid curves) demonstrate a strong curvature due to attenuation correction. In fig. 3.3 it was seen how constant the profiles remain across (and beyond) the boundary of the object so that correcting them for attenuation would be expected to produce the effect observed. The broken line in the figures is a measurement of the line source in air, and the lower, almost superimposed solid line (within the bounds of the object) is the profile of the line source in the cylinder after scatter and attenuation correction. After correction the profiles are similar to that obtained in air, even when the line source is shifted radially.

The opposite extreme in terms of the radionuclide distribution is a uniformly distributed source. The effect on this distribution is shown in fig. 3.10 which shows profiles through the transaxial reconstruction of a cylinder containing a uniformly distributed source with and without scatter correction; both are attenuation corrected using a calculated narrow-beam μ value. The correction is seen to remove the build-up, due to scatter, towards the centre of the object.

The data in fig. 3.11 shows a 3D [^{18}F]-DG scan in a normal volunteer, with and without scatter correction. Scatter correction improves the contrast between grey and white matter. The bottom row shows the result after the subtraction of the scatter corrected reconstructions from the non scatter corrected data. These difference images show the regional effect that scatter correction has had on the data, and bear a remarkable similarity to reconstructed attenuation images, especially the contrast between the air filled sinuses and the brain tissue. The head holder is just visible as well, and emphasises the interaction between scatter and attenuation correction.

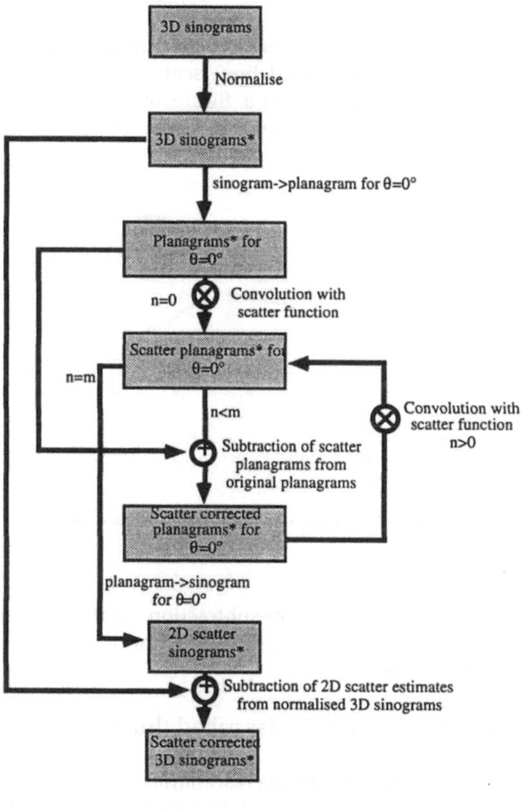

Figure 3.8. The implementation of pre-reconstruction scatter correction using the convolution-subtraction method is illustrated here. Note that normalisation of the emission data is applied before the scatter correction.

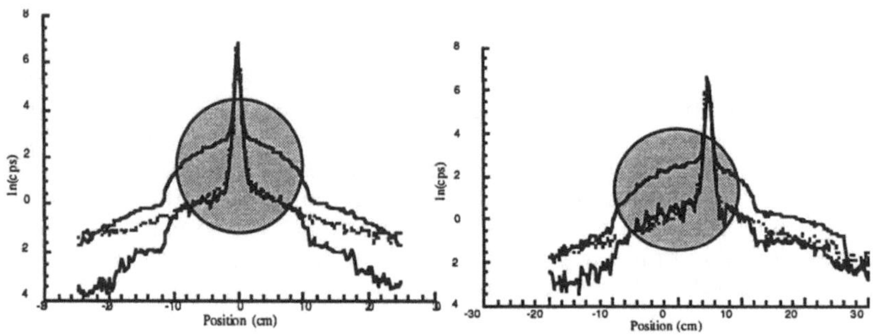

Figure 3.9. Profiles of a positron emitting line source in air (broken line), and in a 20 cm cylinder before (upper solid line) and after (lower solid line) scatter correction with the convolution-subtraction method are shown superimposed on a figure of the cylinder, to scale. The data have been corrected for attenuation, which causes the curvature present in the measurements.

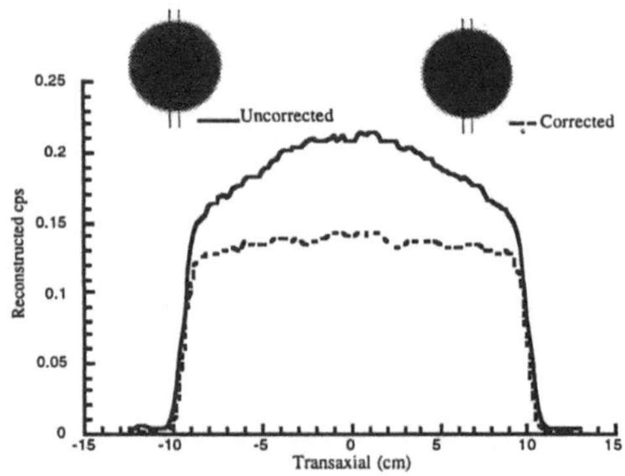

Figure 3.10. Application of the convolution-subtraction scatter correction method to a uniformly distributed source is shown. The solid line is without correction and the broken line after pre-reconstruction scatter correction.

Cherry observed this effect also, which he described thus [Cherry et al., 1993]:

> *"the presence of scatter results in an overestimation of activity in cold regions which have attenuation coefficients similar to water, but an underestimation in regions which have low attenuation coefficients in the range of air. This indicates a preferential redistribution of counts by the filtered backprojection algorithm into areas of high attenuation in the presence of scatter".*

In the regions of the sinuses the subtraction of scatter corrected from non scatter corrected data gives almost zero, indicating that scatter correction had little effect in these low density, air-filled regions. Physically, little scattering would be expected within a region of low density. However, as the coincidence detection method assigns lines-of-response to the pair of detectors which measured the (scattered) event, many lines of response will be assigned incorrectly to projections through the low density region, with probabilities similar to an adjacent, more dense region. Thus, the scatter profile in the projections will hardly be affected by the presence of a small, low density region. However, the attenuation correction factors for this region will be low compared with the surrounding, more dense media. When using a measured transmission scan for attenuation correction, less attenuation correction will be applied to the projections encompassing the low density region, and hence it will be attenuation corrected by a lower factor. When these corrected emission projections are reconstructed, the effect will be to *underestimate* the reconstructed (scatter) count rate from this region. This effect again emphasises the interaction of scatter correction with the other corrections, in this case attenuation.

This scatter correction has used a constant scatter response function, derived from standard objects such as a 20 cm diameter water-filled cylinder, and a global scatter fraction to estimate scatter. Results using this approach for scatter correction in cerebral 3D PET scans have proven to be accurate (see, for example, [Rakshi et al., 1996; Townsend et al., 1996]). However, as Shao has pointed out, this is expected to be less applicable in more heterogeneously attenuating regions of the body such as the thorax. He has suggested that [Shao and Karp, 1995]:

> *"estimating accurately the total scatter fraction is more important than modelling spatially-variant rate constants (scatter functions in our terminology)."*

The results presented in this section would appear to bear this out, and it is a sensible suggestion for further developments in convolution approaches to scatter correction in 3D PET. We have investigated the use of transmission data for estimating scatter fraction per projection more accurately [Bailey et al., 1994], and have demonstrated good results so far in SPECT [Meikle et al., 1991; Meikle et al., 1994]. Whether this will apply as well for 3D PET is still to be determined.

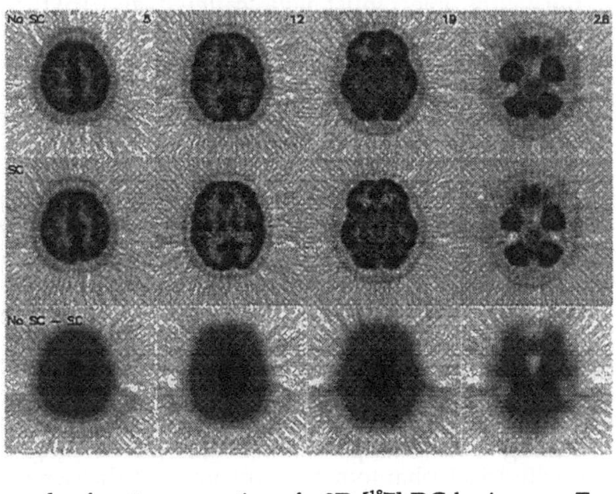

Figure 3.11. An example of scatter correction of a 3D [^{18}F]-DG brain scan. Top row - uncorrected, middle row - corrected for scatter with the convolution-subtraction method, bottom row - the result of subtracting the scatter corrected images from the non scatter corrected images shows the regional differences that the scatter correction has made.

The convolution-subtraction approach has also been applied **after** reconstruction [Lercher et al., 1994]. The method is similar to that described above, where the scatter data are estimated in the 2D planar projection space using data derived from the direct projections (*i.e.*, $\theta \approx 0°$), however, the scatter estimates are reconstructed (rather than subtracted from the measured projections) to give "images" of the "scatter distribution". It is these "scatter images" which are then subtracted from the reconstructed images of the measured data. This raises the question of whether to attenuation correct the measured and "scatter" projections before reconstruction, and if so, with what correction for the scatter data. A number of approaches were investigated in the paper and it was found that attenuation correction applied to the measured data but not the scatter data gave the best compromise. The main advantage of this technique is the computational efficiency with which it can be implemented: while the scatter estimation step will require the same processing time as the other methods, in contrast, the data are then quickly reconstructed with a 2D algorithm rather than subtracted from all projections in the full 3D data set. Thus, after reconstructing the scatter (in 2D) and the emission data (in 3D) all that is required is a simple plane by plane subtraction step.

The approaches that use convolution-subtraction or deconvolution are computationally efficient as they can be implemented on vector processor hardware and the software required for the discrete Fourier transforms (or direct in-place convolution) are widely available. The computational burden can be further reduced by taking advantage of rebinning in the radial and axial dimensions to reduce the data set sizes. Coarse rebinning of this kind is possible because of the low spatial frequency nature of the scatter profiles.

ESTIMATION BY FITTING TO SCATTER OUTSIDE THE OBJECT

This approach to scatter correction is based on (a) the observation that events in the sinogram outside of the source object must have scattered, and, (b) the assumption that the scatter distribution is a low frequency function and relatively insensitive to the activity distribution. The scatter component can thus be estimated by fitting the activity outside the source object with an analytical function (*e.g.*, Gaussian), interpolating the fit inside the object and subtracting the scatter from the measured radioactivity distribution.

The method was originally developed in one dimension (1D), by fitting the tails of the sinogram projection data on a row by row basis. Karp [Karp et al., 1990] implemented the technique on the PENN-PET scanner fitting a parabolic function. Cherry [Cherry et al., 1995]applied this scatter correction technique to PET data from a full ring scanner using a Gaussian fit. The efficacy of the method in improving contrast was verified on a slot phantom, a hot/cold spot phantom and on the 3D Hoffman brain phantom. More recently the method was modified by Stearns [Stearns, 1995] to perform a Gaussian fit in two dimensions on planagrams and the accuracy of correction was verified according to the SNM/NEMA test procedures for evaluating scatter. The method is graphically illustrated in fig. 3.12 using as an example a line source (20 cm long) in the centre of a uniform water-filled cylindrical phantom with an internal diameter and axial length both of 20 cm. Data presented in this section were obtained using the General Electric Advance™ tomograph with a field of view of 55 cm transaxially and 15 cm axially.

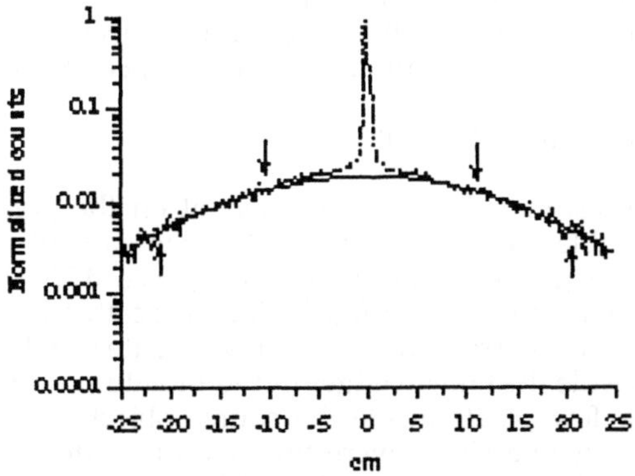

Figure 3.12. Illustration of the Gaussian fitting scatter correction method, applied to a 3D PET scan of a line source in the centre of a 20 cm uniform water phantom. Sinogram profile (dotted line) and fitted Gaussian function (solid line). Up- and down-arrows indicate respectively the starting and ending points used for fitting.

In this implementation, the principal steps in the scatter correction method are as follows:

- smoothing of projection data to reduce noise;
- fitting the tails of the radionuclide distribution outside the source object in projection data by an analytical (Gaussian) function;
- subtracting the estimated scatter component from the measured data.

Situation	Starting Points	Number of Points	Scatter Fraction (%)
A	105 %	40	21
B	90%	40	26
C	105%	15	23
D	90%	15	36

Table 3.1. Scatter fraction determination for a 15 cm uniform phantom. The scatter fraction is affected by the domain of the fit for the profiles. Starting points for fitting are expressed with respect to the effective diameter (15 cm = 100%). Number of points for fitting refer to each side of the profile (pixel size = 2 mm). Scatter fraction is defined by the SNM/NEMA method.

The accuracy of the scatter correction depends on the choice of a set of parameters which should be optimised for each PET scanner and for different radioactivity distributions, in order to accurately estimate scatter components, including:

- the size of the smoothing filter applied to the projection data;

- the starting points of the tails for proper fitting. The starting points of the tails can be selected a few pixels away from the edges of the object, which can be recognised by using the corresponding attenuation map (either calculated or measured);
- the number of points in the tails to fit.

The dependence of the estimated scatter component on the parameters selected for fitting is presented in Table 3.1 and in fig. 3.13, in the case of a uniform cylindrical phantom (15 cm internal diameter and 16 cm high). Fig. 3.13 shows the measured profile and fitted Gaussian functions. In fig. 3.13A the scatter component is estimated by fitting measured data in a correct way, with an adequate number of points for fitting starting a few pixels outside the known edges of the phantom. In fig. 3.13B the starting points have been set a few pixels inside the source object (at 90% of the effective phantom size): this results in a slight overestimation of scatter component within the object and in a slight underestimation outside. When a limited number of points for fitting are used (fig. 3.13C) a good fit is obtained, although the scatter component is slightly overestimated. The combination of these poor assumptions in fig. 3.13D represents an extreme situation (starting points within the object, small number of points for fitting) producing a bad estimate of scatter component.

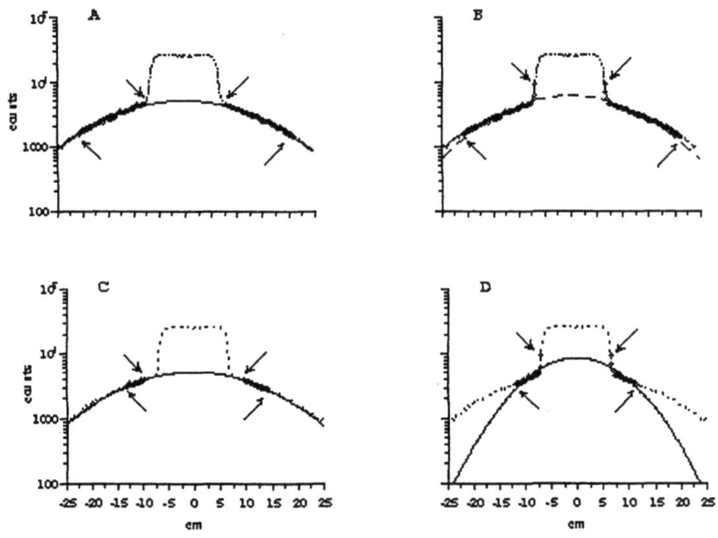

Figure 3.13. Performance of the Gaussian fitting scatter correction method applied to a 15 cm uniform phantom by changing the fitting parameters (see Table 3.1). Measured profile (dotted line) and fitted Gaussian function (solid line). Arrows indicate the range of points used for fitting. (A) Proper choice of the starting points and the number of points for fitting. (B) Proper choice of the number of points for fitting. Starting points are erroneously selected inside the source object. (C) Proper choice of the starting points for fitting. Fitting is performed on a limited number of points. (D) Improper choice of both the starting points and the number of points for fitting. Further studies are required to prove the robustness of the method in a larger variety of asymmetrical radioactivity and object distributions.

An example of the method applied to a 3D [18F]-DG brain study is shown in fig. 3.14 in a comparison of the 3D images without and with scatter correction by the Gaussian fitting method. Fitting parameters were chosen as in fig. 3.13A. A profile through the two images is also shown.

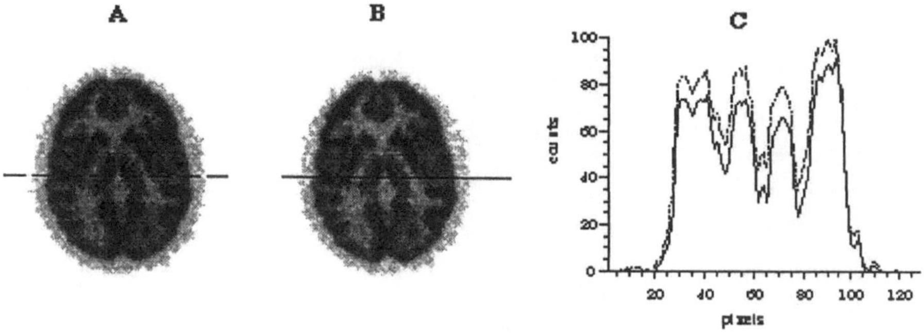

Figure 3.14. Application of the Gaussian fitting scatter correction method to a [18F]FAG brain image. (A) 3D image non-scatter corrected.(B) 3D image scatter corrected by the Gaussian fitting method. (C) Comparison of a profile through image in A (dotted line) and in B (solid line).

One objection raised to the Gaussian fitting scatter correction method is that the assumption that the scatter profile is independent of the radionuclide distribution in the source object might not always be valid. In particular, a Gaussian function might not represent a good model for the scatter component when radioactivity is concentrated in isolated spots, although it may represent a reasonable approximation in a large variety of situations, as shown by Cherry [Cherry et al., 1992].The performance of the method in the case of spheres containing radioactivity embedded in a non-radioactive background is seen in fig. 3.15. The sinogram is shown on the left with lines indicating the positions of the corresponding profiles on the right. A symmetrical scatter distribution outside the source object is seen, in spite of the highly asymmetric distribution inside, suggesting the effectiveness of the method even in this extreme condition.

The main advantages of the Gaussian fitting scatter correction method applied to 3D PET data are:

- the implementation of the method is extremely simple;
- the method does not require supplementary measurements (as in multiple energy window scatter correction methods) nor independent estimations of scatter components (as in methods based on Monte Carlo simulations or convolution-subtraction);
- the correction is extremely computationally efficient and thus rapid;
- the method accounts also for scattered radiation generated from activity outside of the field of view [Cherry et al., 1995]. This is a major point in favour of the technique. It may be that some of the more sophisticated approaches may use this aspect of the method alone to further refine their approaches.

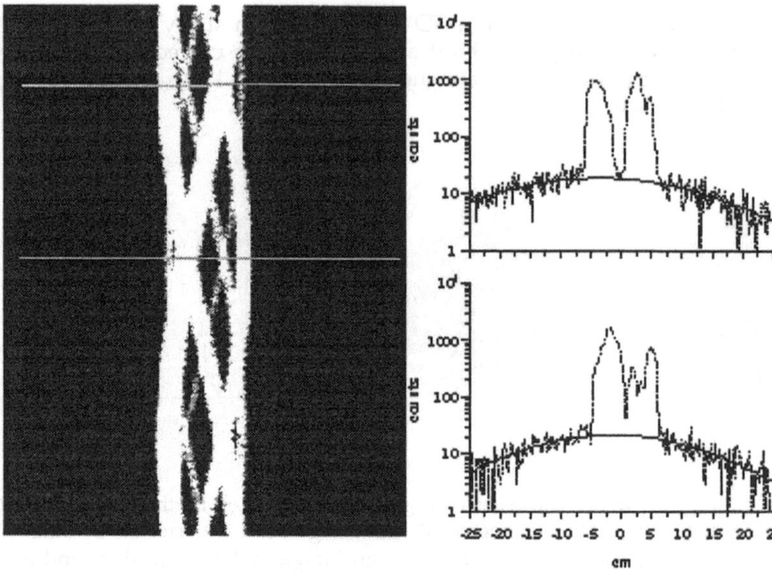

Figure 3.15. Application of the Gaussian fitting scatter correction method to a hot sphere in cold background experiment. Left: sinogram of the 3D PET study, two rows are selected. Right: profiles through the selected row(dotted line) and fitted Gaussian function (solid line)

DIRECT CALCULATION OF SCATTER DISTRIBUTION

This approach is based on the observation that the emission and transmission data contain enough information to accurately compute the distribution of events for which one annihilation photon undergoes a single Compton interaction. This *single scatter* distribution can be used to compute an accurate estimate of the overall scatter distribution for two reasons: single scatters account for roughly 75% of all scattered events and the multiple scatter distribution can be easily approximated from the single scatter distribution [Goggin and Ollinger, 1994]. Barney demonstrated the accuracy of the method for fully 3D imaging by comparing analytic calculations to Monte Carlo studies of several simulated phantom geometries [Barney et al., 1991]. Ollinger showed that accurate scatter estimates could be calculated for slice-collimated PET using measured emission and transmission images [Ollinger, 1991; Ollinger et al., 1993]. Mumcuoglu [Mumcuoglu et al., 1994] applied the same approach to scatter estimation in transmission imaging, and Hiltz [Hiltz et al., 1994] applied it to estimating scatter in PET scanners using multi-wire proportional chambers. This algorithm was extended for use with fully 3D PET and was shown to be computationally feasible for clinical use [Ollinger et al., 1993; Ollinger, 1996; Watson et al., 1996].

Assumptions

1. *Single-scatter approximation.* For the majority of detected scattered events only one of the two photons resulting from an annihilation undergoes a Compton interaction and this photon undergoes a single Compton interaction. This assumption has been shown to be reasonable [Barney et al., 1991; Thompson, 1993]. Monte Carlo studies simulating scans of brain and chest phantoms by a scanner with a 76-cm ring

diameter and a 10-cm axial field-of-view show that 75-80% of scattered coincidences are single scatters, with the exact percentage depending on the source and attenuation geometries.

2. *Multiple scatters.* The implementation by Ollinger [Ollinger, 1996] assumes that the multiple scatter distribution is well modelled as an integral transformation of the single scatter distribution. The magnitude of the kernel is object dependent [Goggin et al., 1994]. The implementation by Watson [Watson et al., 1996] assumes that the multiple scatter distribution differs from the single scatter distribution by a scale factor.

3. *Quantitative emission images.* Emission images accurately reflect the intensity of the annihilation process. The images are corrected for scatter iteratively. It is assumed that corrections for randoms, attenuation, and dead-time are accurate.

4. *Quantitative transmission images.* Transmission images are accurate estimates of the narrow-beam linear attenuation coefficient. They are usually accurate to within 1%.

5. *Detector Efficiency.* The detector efficiency for a scattered coincidence is the same as that for a true coincidence, where detector efficiency is defined to include only effects relating to the detection of incident photons. Geometric effects are incorporated into the single-scatter model and crystal interference effects are incorporated into the normalisation process.

6. *Energy resolution.* Energy resolution is well-modelled as a Gaussian function with a variance determined by the measured energy resolution.

7. *Compton scatter is the dominant interaction.* Photoelectric absorption is rare at the photon energies encountered.

8. *Scatter from outside the field-of-view.* The transmission and emission images are known for most regions that contribute scatter to the data. Scatter originating from regions not sampled by the emission and transmission images has the same spatial distribution as that originating in sampled regions. The estimates for scatter from inside the field-of-view are scaled such that the scatter estimates fit the measured data in measurements that do not sample the body. This implicitly assumes that the distribution of scatter from outside the field-of-view has the same shape as that of scatter from inside the field-of-view.

Computation of the Single Scatter Distribution. In the following section the algorithm set forth in [Ollinger, 1996] is described. See [Watson et al., 1996] for a description of an alternative implementation.

The paths of the annihilation photons for a single scatter are shown by the heavy lines in fig. 3.16. The line-of-flight of the unscattered photon intersects the detector surface at point **A**. The other photon is scattered at a point **S** through an angle ϑ_S and is detected at point **B**. If this photon were not scattered, it would intersect the detector surface at **C**. The scattered coincidence is positioned along the line **AB** of length L. The total scattering angle ϑ_S is decomposed into oblique and transverse components, θ_S and ψ_S, such that θ_S lies in the xy plane.

The idea behind the algorithm is to estimate the number of scattered coincidences along lines-of-response such as **AB** as follows. First, for each scattering point **S** along **AC**, the number of incident photons travelling in the direction ***a*** for which the partner annihilation photon was detected at **A** is calculated. Given this quantity, the total number of photons scattered can be calculated from the linear attenuation coefficient as given by the transmission images. Then the fraction of these scattered toward the detector at **B** can be computed using the Klein-Nishina formula [Klein and Nishina, 1928]. Finally, attenuation along the line **SB** can be calculated from the transmission images. Since the scatter is to be calculated for a specified subset of the lines-of-response in the data, the known variables are the points **A**, **B** and **S**, while the unknown variables are the scattering angle, the angle of incidence at **B**, and the position of the line **SB**.

The mean number of scattered events is found by taking the product of the mean number of incident photons and the joint probability of the following events: (1) of a photon being scattered as it propagates through voxel *s*, (2) of it being scattered towards a detector at **B**, (3) of it not undergoing another interaction before reaching the detector, and (4) of it being detected. Since these are physically independent processes, it can be assumed that each event is statistically independent and the joint probability can be expressed as the product of the marginal probabilities. These probabilities are modelled as follows. The probability of a photon scattering along a path of length Δl is given by $(1-\beta_{sd\theta\psi})$ where β is the survival probability through the voxel at the point specified by $sd\theta\psi$. The probability of a photon scattered at **S** impinging on a detector at **B**, $P_{KN}(l_2,\vartheta_2)$ can be found by integrating the Klein-Nishina formula. The probability of the scattered photon not being attenuated can be found from the transmission images, and is given by $\gamma(l_2,\psi_c,\theta_c,d_s,z_s,E_s)$ where $(\psi_c,\theta_c,d_s,z_s,E_s)$ defines the line along which the scattered photon propagates, l_2 is the distance of the scattering point **S** from the crystal, and E_s is the energy of the scattered photon. The energy spectrum is modelled as a Gaussian function centred at the incident energy of the photon. Integrating this density function yields the probability of an event being accepted by the energy discrimination logic of the scanner. Summing appropriately leads to the expression for the flux of single-scattered photons along the line-of-response ξ_o given by

$$\hat{S}_1(\xi_o)=\frac{4\pi}{\Omega N_\theta}\sum_{\psi\in\Psi}\sum_{\theta\in\Theta}\sum_{d=0}^{D_{max}}\sum_{s=A}^{B}P_E(E_s)\gamma(l_2,\psi_c,\theta_c,d_s,z_s,E_s)P_{KN}(l_2,\vartheta_s)(1-\beta_{sd\theta\psi})$$
$$\times\sum_{l=0}^{s}\eta_{ld\psi}\int_{z_{min}(\psi,l,z_a)}^{z_{max}(\psi,l,z_a)}\lambda_{ld\theta}dz\prod_{i=0}^{l}\beta_{id\theta\psi} \qquad [3.7]$$

where Ω is the solid angle subtended by a single detector ring, N_θ is the number of angular samples in the transverse plane, N_l is the number of oblique angular samples, Θ is a set of transverse angles, and Ψ is a set of oblique angles. The terms in the equation are discussed below.

- *Single-pixel survival probability,* $\beta_{ld\theta\psi}$. This value is calculated from the transmission data. A septa-extended transmission scan is performed and each slice is reconstructed to form a 3D volume of the linear attenuation coefficient at 511 keV sampled at intervals Δl in the *xy* plane and at intervals Δz in the *z* direction. Each value in this volume is scaled by the pixel length, sign-inverted, and exponentiated to form single-pixel survival probabilities. Bilinear interpolation is used to find samples of this volume along the line specified by the angles ψ and θ, the transverse index *d*, and the index corresponding to distance from the detector, *l*.

- *Emission intensity*, $\lambda_{ld\theta}(z)$. The emission intensity is determined as follows. First, sinograms corresponding to straight and cross slices in septa extended scans are extracted from the 3D data set. Straight slices are formed from a direct sinogram and two sinograms with ring difference two. Cross slices are formed from two sinograms with ring difference one and two sinograms with ring difference three. These are then normalised [Ollinger, 1995], corrected for attenuation and summed over angles to yield the desired angular sampling. Scatter is corrected iteratively as discussed subsequently. These images are reconstructed on grid of size Δl in the xy plane and Δz axially.

- *Incidence probability for the unscattered photon*, $\eta_{ls\psi}$. This probability models two effects: the probability of a photon emitted at a distance *l* and angle ψ from a detector being detected, and the probability of the partner to an unscattered, detected photon impinging on the scattering voxel. Since these are separate physical processes, they can be assumed to be statistically independent. The probability of the first effect is simply the ratio of the solid angle subtended by a detector at distance *l*, *i.e.*, Ω_u , to 4π. The second effect arises because the implementation implicitly assumes that photons propagate along a path with parallel sides in the transverse plane. However, suppose that for voxel at a distance *l* from the detector, photons travelling away from the detector diverge at an angle given by θ′ and that for a voxel at **S**, the detector subtends an angle θ''. Then, the fraction of photons emitted at the first voxel incident at **S** can be approximated by θ'/θ. The overall probability is given by

$$\eta_{l\psi}=\frac{\Omega_u(l)\theta''}{4\pi\theta'} \qquad [3.8]$$

- *Probability of scattering to a given detector*, $P_{KN}(l_2,\vartheta_s)$. This probability is computed by integrating the Klein-Nishina formula.

- *Attenuation of the scattered photon*, $\gamma(l_2,\psi_c,\theta_c,d_s,z_s,E_s)$. The attenuation along the path of the scattered photon is calculated as follows. First, two tables are constructed: one of attenuation at 511 keV, $\gamma(l_2,\psi_c,\theta_c,d_s,z_s,E_s=511)$, and the other, $\rho(E_S)=\mu_w(E_S)/\mu_w(E_{511})$, the ratio of the attenuation coefficient of water at energy E_S to the attenuation coefficient of water at 511 keV. Since Compton scatter dominates at the energies of interest in biological tissues, and since the component of the attenuation coefficient due to Compton scatter depends solely on electron density, the attenuation coefficient at energy E_S can be approximated by $\mu(E_S)=\rho(E_S)/\mu(E_{511})$. The attenuation factor is exponentially related to the linear attenuation coefficient and $\rho(E_S)$ is independent of position, so the attenuation factor can be written as

$$\gamma\left(l_2,\psi_c,\theta_c,d_s,z_s,E_S\right)=\gamma\left(l_2,\psi_c,\theta_c,d_s,z_s,E_s=511\right)^{\rho\left(E_S\right)} \qquad [3.9]$$

- *Probability of being accepted by energy discrimination*, $P_E(E_S)$. The measured energy is modelled as a normally-distributed random variable with the mean equal to the energy of the incident photon and the variance at energy *E*, σ_E^2, determined by the energy-resolution of the detectors using the relation

$$\sigma_E^2 = \sigma_{511}^2 \sqrt{E_S/511} \qquad [3.10]$$

where σ_{511}^2 is the energy resolution at 511 keV and E_S is the energy of the scattered photon [Thompson, 1993]. The probability of an incident photon with energy E_S being accepted is found by integrating the normal distribution. A single energy resolution is assumed for all detectors.

- *Solid angle, Ω.* The scanner does not measure the true intensity of the emission process, but rather observes it through an aperture determined by the solid angle Ω subtended by the detector rings. Since the scatter estimate is a linear function of the reconstructed images, it must be scaled by the ratio $4\pi/\Omega$.

Multiple Scatters. The multiple scatter distribution is modelled as the convolution of the single-scatter distribution with a one-dimensional Gaussian kernel [Goggin et al., 1994]. This model is motivated by several considerations. First, the multiple scatter distribution is much more similar to the single-scatter distribution than the total scatter distribution is to the true event distribution, so a convolutional model relating multiple scatters to single scatters should be more accurate than a convolutional model relating total scatters to true events. Second, the model is easily implemented and can be quickly calculated. And finally, multiple scatters are a relatively small fraction of the total number of scattered events, so errors in their calculation are less important than errors in the calculation of the single scatters. The FWHM of this kernel was shown to be relatively fixed for a given ring diameter. The magnitude was found to vary with the path length through the object being imaged and can be estimated from the transmission images. For a typical brain study, approximately 20% of the detected scattered events are multiple scatters. This percentage increases to 25% for a line-source centred in a chest-sized phantom. It has a value of 23% for a uniform chest phantom.

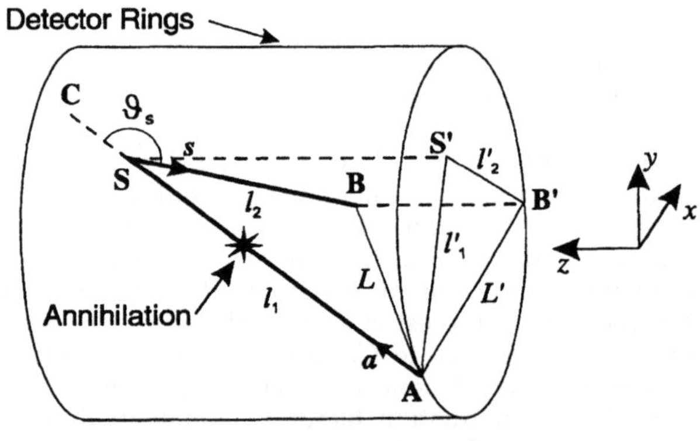

Figure 3.16. Three dimensional view of a scattered event that has undergone a single Compton interaction.

Iteration. The algorithm given by equation 3.7 requires knowledge of the intensity of the emitted photons. This intensity is not known. Rather, the measured sinograms represent the sum of true and scattered events. True sinograms are iteratively computed from the measured data using the method of successive substitutions.

Implementation. The overall algorithm is implemented as shown in the following pseudocode:

```
Extract direct-plane emission and transmission sinograms

Reconstruct transmission images

For (number of iterations)

        Reconstruct emission images

        Estimate scatter for direct planes

        Correct direct-plane sinograms

        Reconstruct emission images

Estimate scatter for direct and oblique angles

Correct 3D emission sinograms
```

Evaluation. Evaluations of this method using phantoms and human studies [Ollinger, 1996; Watson et al., 1996] show that accuracy equivalent to that of septa-extended imaging can be achieved if the activity outside the field-of-view is either much smaller than that inside the field-of-view or has the same spatial distribution.

A qualitative assessment of the accuracy of the method is shown by the following study. The chest was simulated by an elliptical phantom (Data Spectrum model 2230) with major and minor axes of 30.5 and 22 cm respectively containing anthropomorphic lung inserts (Data Spectrum model 3025). It contained two 6-cm diameter spheres filled with ^{18}F at concentrations of 12.5% and 25% of background. The background contained 100 kBq of ^{18}F. This phantom was scanned in two configurations: with air-filled lungs and containing a Teflon spine insert, and with cold, water-filled lungs and no spine insert. It was scanned with septa-retracted and with septa-extended for each configuration. The duration of the scans simulated a three-fold dose reduction with the septa retracted. For the air-filled lung configuration 386 million counts were collected with septa retracted and 195 million with septa extended. For the water-filled lung configuration these numbers fell to 323 million and 155 million counts respectively. Transmission and blank scans were one hour long.

Results of this study shown in fig. 3.17 suggest that the accuracy of the corrected fully 3D images is equivalent to the septa-extended images, even in highly heterogeneous attenuating media. Quantitative results from phantom studies and humans [Ollinger, 1996; Watson et al., 1996] support this conclusion in terms of absolute accuracy, uniformity, and assessments of human studies.

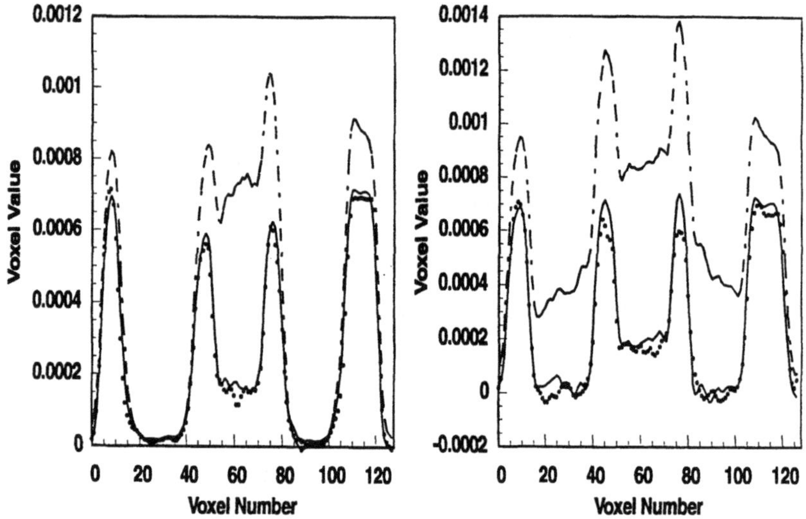

Figure 3.17. Profiles through the chest phantom with air-filled lungs (left) and water-filled lungs (right). The dashed line represents the uncorrected 3D images, the solid line the scatter-corrected 3D images, and the closed circles represent the 2D images.

Summary. Direct calculation of the scatter distribution is quantitatively accurate if scatter from outside the field-of-view is either low in magnitude or similar in shape to the scatter from inside the field-of-view. Scatter from outside the field-of-view can be directly taken into account by acquiring short, auxiliary scans adjacent to the axial volume being investigated. Indeed, the phantom studies reported in [Ollinger, 1996] used this approach. These data are naturally available for whole-body imaging. However, this method would be of doubtful utility if the isotope has a short half-life or has rapid uptake relative to the scanning interval.

This method's greatest advantage is that it accurately accounts for variations in the attenuating medium. This should make it particularly well suited for studies in the chest, particularly those where the liver is either relatively cold or distant from the field-of-view. Although it is accurate in studies of the head, it might not have a clear-cut advantage over simpler, less computationally intensive methods.

Scatter from outside the field of view

As we have seen, correction for scatter coincidences may be effected by either energy-based, convolution (integral-transform), or direct calculation methods. The latter two will be plagued by limitations in dealing with scatter from outside the field of view. As seen earlier in fig. 3.5, the scattering in the axial dimension is reasonably constant. The consequence of this is that there will be scatter *into* the coincidence field of view (defined by the axial length of the scanner, see fig. 3.18) from outside the region under study. These are true coincidence events as they arise from the same positron annihilation, however, the only way geometrically that they can be detected within the field of view is if one or both have been scattered. The energy-based approaches, which can accommodate out of field scatter, will probably require more energy information than is provided by a single "scatter" window, and, ideally, a full energy spectrum would be used. This places enormous demands on data acquisition and computation hardware. Improved energy resolution from better scintillation materials would help, but energy resolution is probably not going to exceed 8%-10% FWHM at 511 keV. Therefore in 3D PET, scatter will always be present and methods for dealing with it will be required. The incorporation of transmission data into the non energy-based methods may help in improving their accuracy.

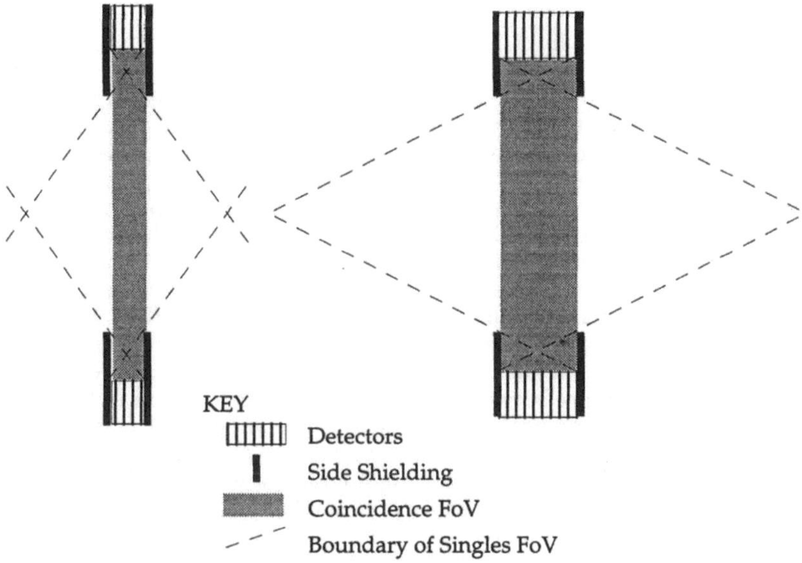

Figure 3.18. Cross-sectional diagram (to scale) of the first whole body 2D/3D PET scanner (ECAT 951R) (left) which has a 102 cm diameter detector ring, 10.8 cm axial field of view, and side shielding which left a patient aperture of approximately 62 cm. The EXACT 3D (right) is the first full-time 3D BGO based full ring tomograph. It has an 86 cm diameter detector ring, 23.4 cm axial field of view, and side shielding that leaves a patient aperture also of approximately 62 cm. This has a dramatic effect on the field of view for single events that can irradiate the detectors. This increases dead time as well as scattered and random coincidences relative to the well-shielded detectors in the 951R. (Both diagrams to same scale).

A study of the impact of scatter from outside the field of view on quantitative parameter estimates in cerebral studies has been reported [Townsend et al., 1996]. Using ^{11}C-Flumazenil, scatter correction with both the dual energy window and convolution-subtraction methods was found to remove bias in the parameter estimates due to scatter and return the values similar to those obtained in 2D scans (but with less uncertainty because of the higher quality of the 3D scans). In phantom studies in this report, the dual energy window approach corrected more accurately for scattered events from outside the field of view, however, the authors concluded that this was unlikely to be a major problem for cerebral studies, particularly as the axial field of view of current tomographs can encompass the whole brain unlike previous devices. It does remain a challenging issue for thoracic and abdominal studies, though, and it is likely that scattered photon energy information will prove useful in accurately dealing with scatter from outside the field of view irrespective of the method used to estimate the scattered coincidences. The trend today is to increase the axial field of view of 3D PET systems and this leads to a greater acceptance of events from outside the coincidence field of view. These events will contribute unwanted scattered and random coincidences to the measurements.

Normalisation Methods for 3D PET

APPROACHES TO NORMALISATION

Normalisation of the 3D scan data, *i.e.*, the correction for non-uniformity of detector response and corrections related to the geometry of the scanner, has received relatively less attention than scatter correction until recently. The first multi-slice 3D data acquired and reconstructed on a full ring BGO block detector tomograph used a blank scan obtained from a low activity rotating rod source to generate a normalisation for all lines of response [Townsend et al., 1989]. This is an example of what can be termed a *direct method* of obtaining a normalisation, *i.e.*, the data acquired for the normalisation are "inverted" to provide a correction factor directly from the measured data, after a global normalisation to give an overall gain of unity. Subsequent to this, *indirect methods* were developed which used 2D data sets to model individual detector responses rather than coincidence events and the product of any two then produces an estimate of the sensitivity for a line of response between the two detectors [Casey and Hoffman, 1986; Chesler and Stearns, 1990]. The use of 2D data for generating a 3D normalisation was born of necessity as the radioactive sources available were intended for use in 2D normalisation, and as such had prohibitively high count rates when used in 3D [Cherry et al., 1991; Defrise et al., 1991]. There are a number of criticisms of the indirect approaches, however, which include:

- if the normalisation is acquired with transmission ring or rod sources, the location of the sources relative to the detectors are very different to that when imaging an object in the centre of the tomograph (this applies to both 2D and 3D acquisitions) [Kinahan et al., 1995];

- f it is acquired in 2D mode with septa in place in the field of view, the response of the detectors is very different to the 3D situation due to the large shadowing effect that the septa have on the blocks (this applies irrespective of the source, whether rotating rods, uniform cylinder, or plane source);

- it is difficult to model all effects accurately as it is possible that corrections will vary with both azimuthal angle(ϕ) and polar angle(θ), as well as potential interactions between these;

- if a uniform cylinder is used in 3D the scatter present may distort the normalisation.

Plane sources have been suggested as the ideal geometry for PET normalisation [Hoffman et al., 1989; Stazyk et al., 1994]. Recently, a practical, low-cost alternative to the conventional solid plane source, which uses a moving line source to emulate a plane source, has been developed [Bailey and Jones, 1995]. In the following section some of the documented causes of nonuniformity in 2D and 3D PET measurements are described, before a discussion of various strategies that have been employed to deal with these.

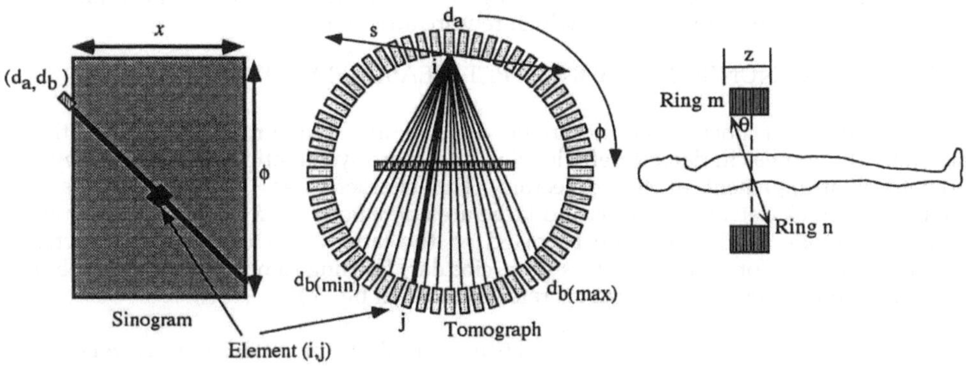

Figure 3.19. The coordinate system for the calculation of the 3D normalisation factors is shown in the diagram

Choice of Source for Normalizing 3D PET. The sources which have been used for normalizing 3D PET systems include:

- plane source using ^{68}Ge [Stazyk et al., 1994];
- uniform 20 cm diameter cylinder, usually containing ^{68}Ge [Kinahan et al., 1995];
- ^{68}Ge transmission scanning rod sources in 2D [Defrise et al., 1991];
- ^{68}Ge transmission scanning rod sources in 3D [Casey et al., 1995];
- a line source of ^{68}Ge which oscillates across the transaxial field of view, emulating a plane source [Bailey et al., 1996].

Bearing in mind the above concerns, a number of these reports have found that transmission scanning rod sources can be used for deriving the normalization factors [Casey et al., 1995] and that little difference is observed between rod sources and a uniform cylinder [Kinahan et al., 1995]. Dead time remains the main problem in using rod sources intended for 2D for 3D acquisition of normalization data. Casey have isolated the normalization into different components [Casey et al., 1995] to maintain flexibility in applying this with different acquisition strategies, as modern 3D PET systems allow great freedom in the configuration and on-line rebinning of the projection data to restrict the size of the data sets. This method overcomes the need to keep different normalisations for each different acquisition configuration. It is clear that using a uniform cylinder for the normalization data will include a significant amount of scatter in this measurement; what is not clear, however, is whether this is a good thing or not. Scatter in the measurement means that the energy spectra from the detectors will be similar to that from a subject having a scan. The consequences of a large number of scattered coincidences being recorded in the normalization data has not been studied in great detail.

It seems that the best approach to normalization of 3D PET data is to use data acquired in 3D, rather than 2D. The best source geometry and the method of calculating the corrections are not as clear. The following section discusses different normalization effects in the data from ring systems which require attention.

SOURCES OF NONUNIFORMITY IN 3D PET MEASUREMENTS

The components of normalisation can be divided into two broad categories: those caused by differences in detector efficiencies, and more systematic effects caused by the geometrical arrangement of the detectors. The characteristics of these effects are different for block detector systems and large area detectors, such as gamma cameras in coincidence mode. Little has been reported on the latter. The next section describes some of the effects for block detectors on a circular, full ring tomograph (ECAT 953B). All symbols and reference coordinates refer to those in fig. 3.19.

Detector Efficiency Non-Uniformity Correction. The **detector efficiency correction** is calculated from data which uniformly irradiates all detectors (such as a uniform cylinder or a plane source). For each individual detector it is assumed that all lines of response will have approximately the same coincident photon flux, and that most fan sums do not vary greatly from the average fan sum [Casey et al., 1986; Chesler et al., 1990] . The individual detector efficiency E for crystal *i* in ring *m* is given by:

$$\langle E(i,m) \rangle = \frac{\sum_{x=x_{min},\, \phi=\phi_{min}}^{x_{max},\, \phi_{max}} S(x,\phi,m,n)}{\frac{1}{N}\sum_{n=1}^{N} \sum_{x=x_{min},\, \phi=\phi_{min}}^{x_{max},\, \phi_{max}} S(x,\phi,m,n)} \qquad [3.11]$$

where $S(x,\phi,m,n)$ is the sensitivity of a line of response for the sinogram element $s(x,\phi)$ between rings m and n, and there are N detectors in total. The impact of the detector efficiency correction factors is shown in fig. 3.20 where the correction factors calculated from the above equation have been applied to the assembled data from a plane source acquisition. Each diagonal line is formed by the responses measured between a single detector on one side of the ring and the fan it forms coincidences with on the opposite side. A diagonal line of low response is therefore due to a single detector having a low efficiency.

Geometric Profile Correction. There is a decrease in count rate towards the centre of the projection in a circular ring scanner due to the increasing collinearity between the lines of response and the gaps between the detectors in the block, and the decreasing centre-to-centre spacing between detectors towards the edge of the transverse field of view due to the curvature of the ring. The transaxial **geometric profile** [Bergström et al., 1982] as a function of ring difference (detector ring combinations in the polar angle θ) was calculated from the equation:

$$G(s,m,n) = \frac{1}{N_\phi} \sum_{\phi=1}^{N_\phi} S(x,\phi,m,n) \qquad [3.12]$$

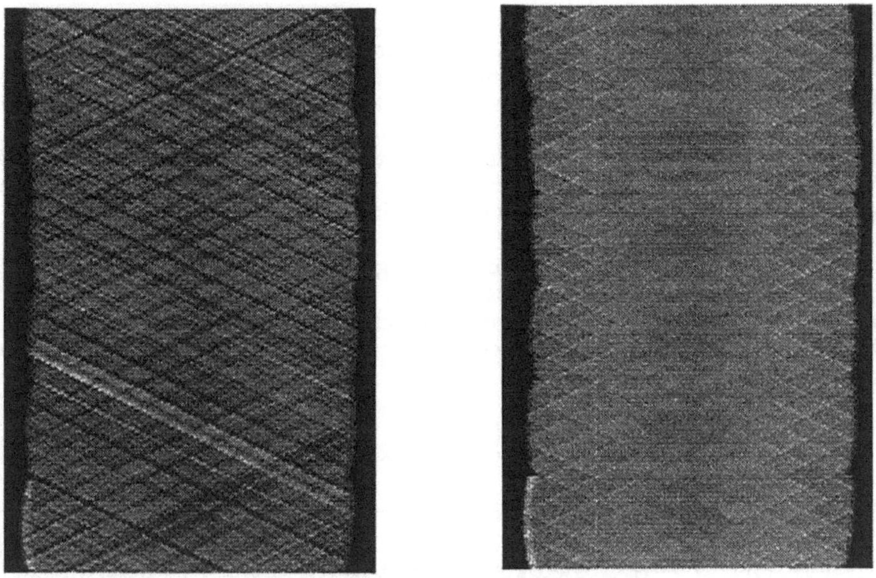

Figure 3.20. Data from a plane source acquisition are shown on the left and the result after the calculation of, and correction for, detector efficiencies is displayed on the right. The decreased values towards the centre on the corrected sinogram clearly demonstrate the need for the ring geometric profile correction.

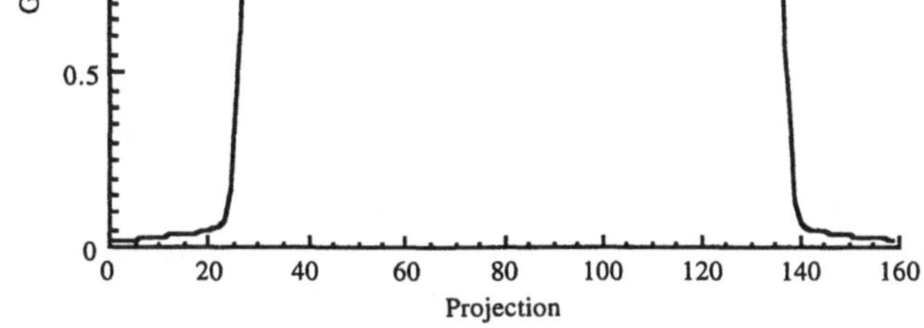

Figure 3.21. The geometric profile for the sum of all direct planes (m = n) is shown.

where N_ϕ is the number of radial projections (rows in the sinogram).The profile is simply the sum over columns of the data in a sinogram. A typical geometric profile for a ring tomograph is shown in fig. 3.21. For tomographs with relatively small maximum polar acceptance angle (typical axial field of view less than 15 cm) and therefore a small range of oblique projection angles this profile has been found to be constant for all rings with the same ring difference and over all ring differences. The effect on the reconstructions of this "hole" towards the centre of the acquisition matrix will be demonstrated later, but may help to explain why the increased magnitude of scatter did not appear at first to be an obvious problem in early 3D reconstructions.

Crystal Interference. **Crystal interference** is the geometric response profile of a given detector with each detector in the opposing block [Casey et al., 1995]. This is a pattern which is repeated for that detector in every block, and so steps in units equal to the number of detectors radially in the block (8 for the ECAT 953B and 951R). It is given by the following:

$$X(x,k,m,n) = \frac{1}{N_s} \sum_{\phi=1}^{N_s} s(x,k+(\phi-1)N_{det},m,n) \qquad [3.13]$$

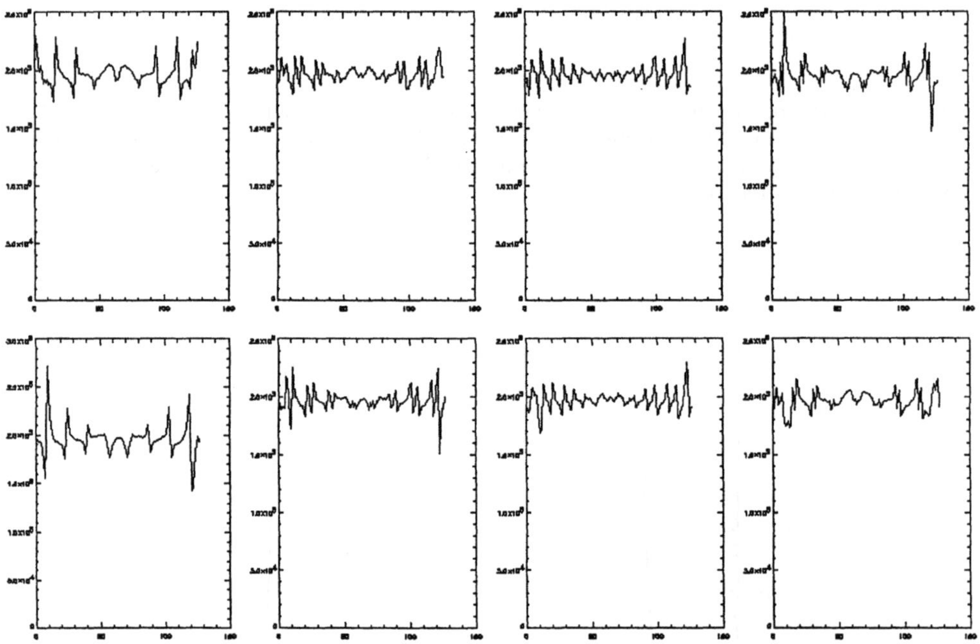

Figure 3.22. The crystal interference profiles for all rings with $\Delta p=0$ for each of the 8 detectors radially are shown. The x axis is the projection dimension (x_r). These factors are consistent from ring to ring on the ECAT 953B. Each graph corresponds to one of the eight detectors 1-8 (from top left to bottom right) in an ECAT 95x series block. The relative scaling of the profiles is arbitrary.

where N_{det} are the number of detectors radially in one block, $N_s = N_\phi/N_{det}$ are the number of sinogram rows (s) to average together, and k is the position of the detector in the block, given by $k = \mathrm{mod}(i, N_{det})$, such that $1 \le k \le N_{det}$. The crystal interference profiles for each of the eight detectors from the direct sinograms (*i.e.*, m = n) are shown in fig. 3.22. Again, these profiles are fairly constant for each detector position in the block over increasing ring differences.

The overall normalisation factors are given by combining each of the above:

$$N(x,\phi,m,n)=\frac{1}{[(\langle E(i,m)\rangle\langle E(j,n)\rangle)G(x,m,n)X(x,k,m,n)]} \quad [3.14]$$

where one or all of the corrections may be omitted. When the geometric factors are combined a geometric correction sinogram can be formed and this is shown in fig. 3.23. In the following results a 20 cm diameter cylinder containing a solution of ^{68}Ge was measured for 12 hours in an ECAT 953B tomograph, accumulating a total of 2.6×10^9 counts to give a high statistics data set on which to assess the impact of the various corrections. It was possible to isolate the effects documented above, and in this way, examine the effect of successively adding each correction.

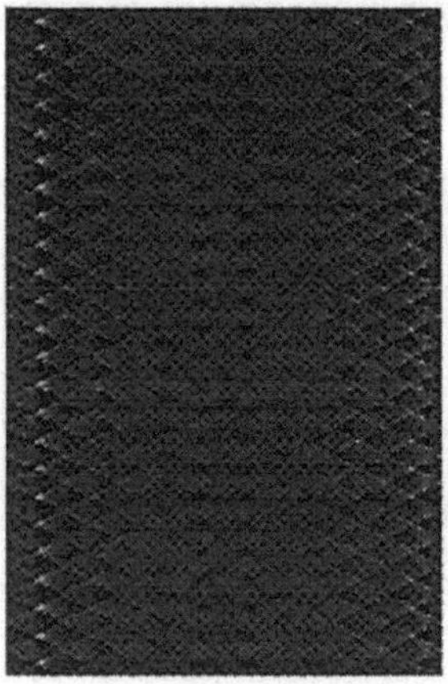

Figure 3.23. The combination of all of the geometric corrections is shown displayed as a sinogram. The bright and dark "corners" of the diamonds towards the edge of the field of view correspond to the peaks and troughs that are seen in the crystal interference profiles, especially for detectors 4 and 5.

This is contrasted with the simplest direct method for normalization, *i.e.*, calculating $1/(x,\phi)$ for each element in the plane source data. In this method no assumptions are made about the data and the correction factor is simply the inverse of the count in each pixel globally normalized for unity gain.

Effects on Reconstructed Images. The effects on the reconstructed images of the uniform cylinder for each of the different corrections are shown in fig. 3.23. All data were reconstructed using the reprojection algorithm with ramp filter and calculated attenuation correction. The scatter correction was the convolution-subtraction method. The first effect observed in general is that the scatter in the image "offsets" the relative decrease seen towards the centre of the reconstruction in all conditions. This is especially well demonstrated in fig. 3.24a and 3.24b. Application of a single geometric profile correction (fig. 3.24c) effectively removes this. A residual ring artefact is still seen at roughly half the radius of the cylinder, as well as a small hole in the centre of the image matrix. The addition of the crystal interference profile (fig. 3.24d) reduces both of these effects, although they are still present. It is a subtle effect only visible on high count density images, and would not be expected to be noticeable on a typical human study. The direct normalisation (fig. 3.24e) appears to correct for all of the geometric effects identified, but produces an artefactual increase at the centre of the scanner, where small inaccuracies are amplified in the reconstruction process. The origin of this artefact is yet to be determined.

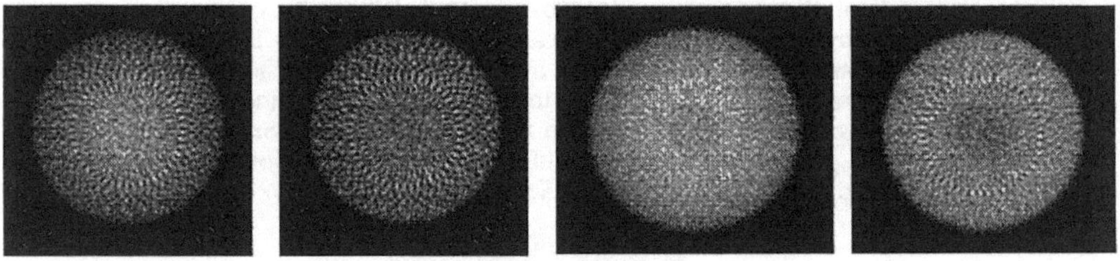

(a) No corrections *(b) Detector efficiency correction only*

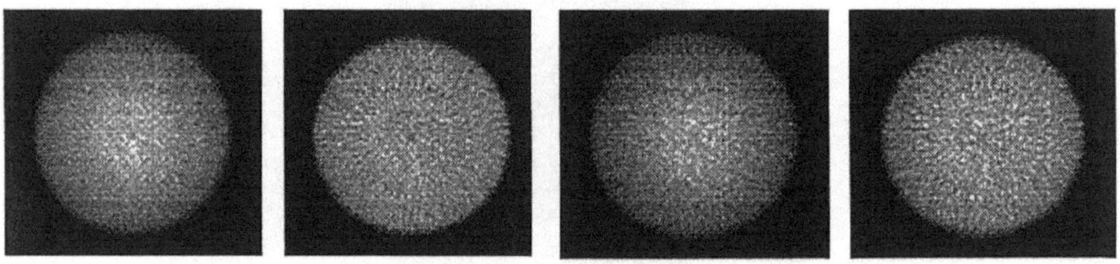

(c) Detector efficiency and geometric corrections *(d) Detector efficiency, geometric and crystal interference corrections*

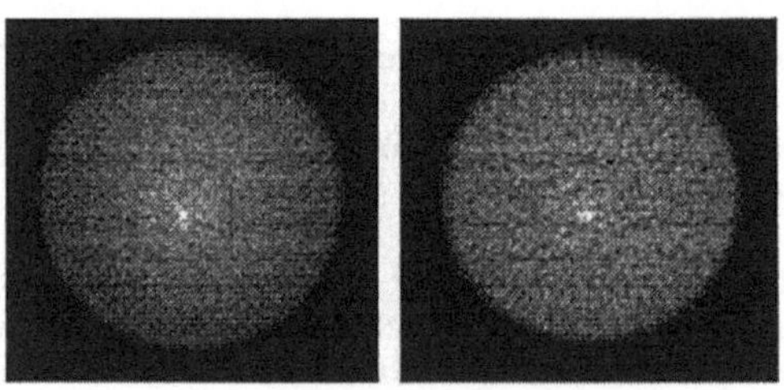

(e) Direct normalisation from the inverted plane source data

Figure 3.24. The effect on the reconstruction of a uniform cylinder of the various corrections is shown. All reconstructions have used a calculated attenuation correction. In each case the image on the left is not corrected for scatter and the image on the right has been scatter corrected before reconstruction.

It can be seen that failing to correct for the variations in sensitivity between detectors has a dramatic impact on the quality of the data produced. The simplest strategy for normalisation may be to record plane source data of sufficiently high quality that it can be used *directly* for normalisation of the data, thus negating the need to model the various aspects studied separately above. This is attractive as it makes no assumptions about the factors that need to be corrected for, and has been shown to remove the majority of artefacts that were seen here. It does, however, introduce a small artefact located at the central axis of the scanner which, to date, is unexplained. It may be that because the source that was used (moving line source emulating a plane source) provides virtually scatter-free data there is a difference in either the energy spectrum per detector or the individual efficiencies of the detectors compared with an emission acquisition in which a significant number of events are scattered. Any slight discrepancies here will be accentuated at the centre of the scanner by the backprojection process.

The direct normalisation approach should provide a gold standard for normalisation, but has the drawback that for 3D data it may be excessive, as high counting statistics are required at a number of projection angles. The effects related to geometry and block patterns seen here would not be expected to vary during the life of a tomograph and may require measurement once only at initial commissioning. A simple detector efficiency correction using either a plane source or cylinder could then be performed on a routine basis.

When using *indirect* 'modelling' approaches for normalisation, the circular sampling geometry leaves a region of relatively decreased count rate in the centre of the image, which is accentuated by scatter correction. Early studies with 3D PET demonstrated less scatter than might have been expected in the reconstructed data, when physical measurements and simulation suggested a much higher component should be present. The cause was probably that the lack of a geometric correction was being offset by the extra scattered events in the reconstructed data. The interaction between scatter and normalisation in 3D PET is strong, and methods for studying the effects in isolation are essential. The corrections discussed here were found to be relatively constant over different rings and ring differences, however the ECAT 953B tomograph has a relatively restricted polar acceptance angle. In the reconstructions here, a single geometric and crystal interference profile was used, derived from all data and ring differences. This may not be appropriate for tomographs with larger axial acceptance angles. One of the assumptions in the calculation of detector efficiency from the fan sums (the sum of counts for one detector in coincidence with all of the detectors on the opposing side of the ring, or 'fan') in the indirect method is the approximate equivalence of the fan sum totals for different detectors. The data in fig. 3.19 demonstrates a fairly large range (~50%-150%) and fractional standard deviation (~10%-13%) in count rates which may invalidate this approach.

ASSESSING NORMALIZATION

It would be highly desirable to have a quantitative metric with which to assess normalization. The usual uniformity measures (*e.g.*, NEMA, EEC) calculate the mean and standard deviation for regions of interest (*e.g.*, 1 cm^2 regions) in reconstructed images. For geometric effects such as those present in the above reconstructions these will obviously be insensitive. The most accurate assessment would be one that was oriented to examining circular differences in images, for ring-based systems. Some authors have limited themselves to considering the total counts in the projections (graphing sinogram or projection number against total counts in the projection). Clearly, the best place to assess the impact of the effects seen above is in the reconstructed image, as the filtered-backprojection reconstruction procedure is known to amplify small, systematic non-uniformities towards the centre of the reconstructed volume. This is dramatically demonstrated in the following example. The effect of a systematic nonuniformity of 2% below the true count is shown in fig. 3.25. The data that were used to derive this graph were from a synthesised data set, with noise added, and in which 2 columns in the sinogram had the count rate decreased by 2% of the true value. The data were reconstructed without normalization or attenuation correction and the mean count in the ring artefact induced by this process found.

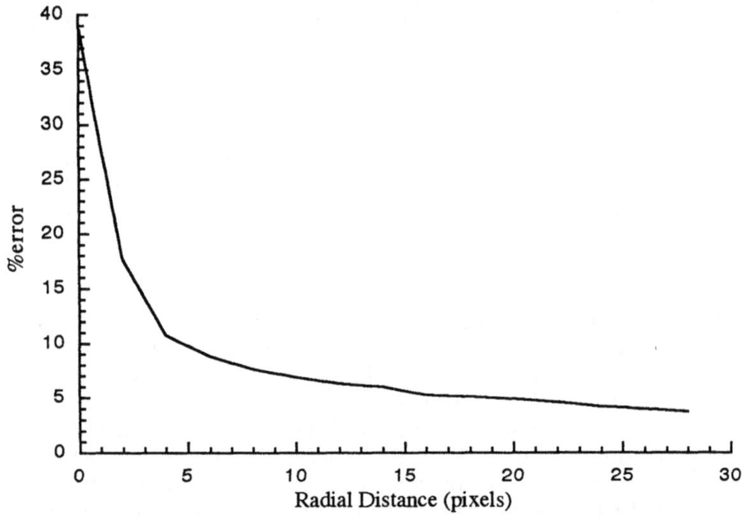

Figure 3.25. The impact in terms of a reduction in reconstructed count rate due to a -2% nonuniformity in the sinogram is shown as a function of radial distance from the centre of the sinogram matrix. At the centre the reconstructed count is reduced by ~40%. As the nonuniformity is moved away from the centre of the matrix it produces a "ring artefact" of diminishing impact.

The 2% nonuniformity produced almost a 40% decrease in the reconstructed value when the artificially decreased projections were in the middle of the sinogram; this drops off rapidly as the defect was moved off centre. This would strongly suggest that assessing the images is a more rigorous test than assessing the projection data.

One approach to quantifying the artefacts of normalization in 3D PET that has been reported [Bailey et al., 1996] uses an adapted form of the parameter "integral uniformity" defined in the NEMA gamma camera test procedures [NEMA, 1986]. The mean and standard deviation was calculated within annular regions of interest in the reconstructed images. This, in effect, is simply replacing square regions of interest with annular ones. As the effects observed are related to the geometry of the scanner rather than the object, the centre of the scanner (*i.e.*, pixel (64,64) in the 128 x 128 reconstructed images) was taken as the centre for the regions. Regions of interest were defined for annular rings calculated at one pixel radial increments over 360 degrees for all pixels contained within the boundary of the cylinder. For each plane (p) and annular ring (r) the mean ($\varepsilon(r,p)$) and coefficient of variation ($CoV(r,p)$) of the annular region was determined. No correction was made for the increasing number of pixels in the sample with increasing radius. The values were then averaged over all planes and the maximum and minimum average $\varepsilon(r)$ found to measure the absolute *nonuniformity index* (NUI).

The absolute nonuniformity index for the radial mean count measures the largest variation in the mean value between the annuli. The nonuniformity index for the plane-averaged $CoV(r)$ is determined in an identical manner from the coefficient of variation values, and is a measure of the amount of variation that exists *within* an annulus; the circular pattern that persists in the images in fig. 3.23 would be expected to give a high coefficient of variation.

Fig. 3.26 shows the mean radial count for two extreme situations: the cylinder with no normalisation applied (fig. 3.23a) and with all corrections applied (fig. 3.23d). These data are the average of the results for all planes. Without normalisation the mean count is greater at the centre and decreases towards the edge of the cylinder, whereas the data with all corrections is generally lower (due to scatter removal) and more uniform radially across the cylinder. The nonuniformity index is a measure of this variability. Fig. 3.27 shows the radial coefficient of variation for the same two conditions (*i.e.*, no normalisations, and all corrections). This parameter should demonstrate "ring" effects, especially the circular pattern.

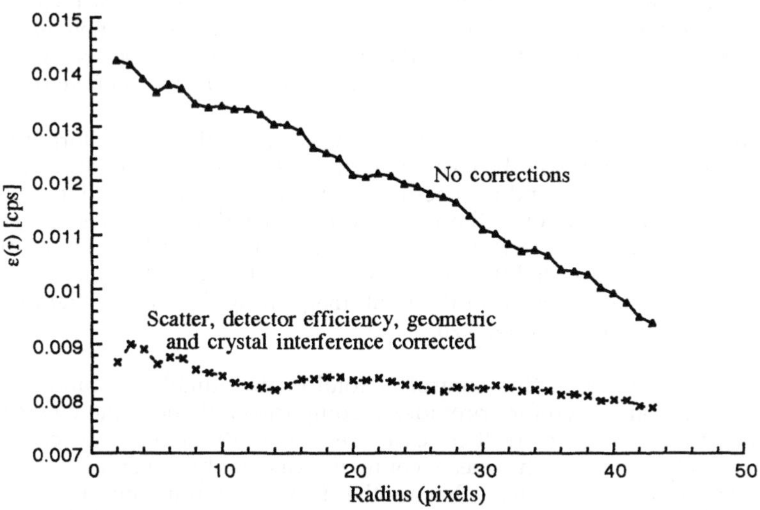

Figure 3.26. The graph shows the mean counts in the annular regions of interest in the reconstructed images for the extreme conditions of no normalisation (Fig 3.23a), and all corrections (Fig 3.23d). The maximum and minimum are used to quantify the nonuniformity index of variability in the reconstruction.

In this case the reconstruction without any normalisation is lower at the centre than the case with all the corrections applied. This is due to the increased scatter build-up at this location. However, the $CoV(r,p)$ soon increases dramatically. The data with all corrections are again far more consistent across the object. Both data sets show the circular pattern due to the ring, which is far more marked in the data with no corrections.

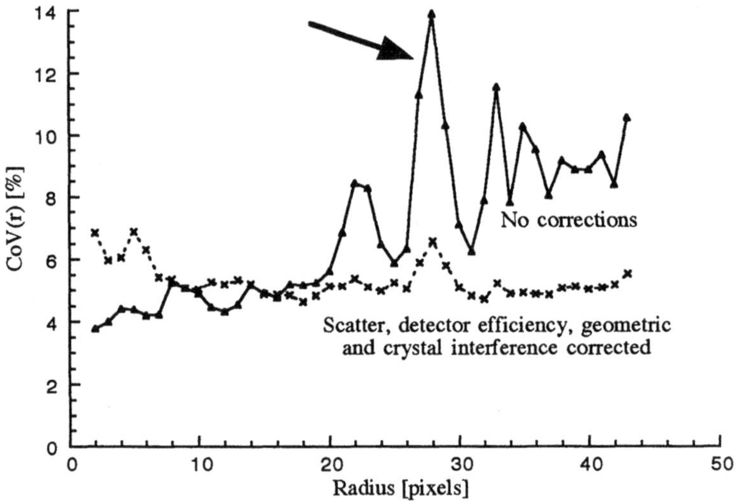

Figure 3.27. The coefficient of variation averaged over all planes is shown as a function of radial distance in the uniform cylinder. The arrow indicates the location of the circular artefact pattern, but shows that the coefficient of variation is more constant after the normalisations have been applied. These data are used to compute the nonuniformity index.

The data in these graphs are reduced to a single figure, the nonuniformity index, by measuring the greatest range in the individual ring values. The nonuniformity indices for the mean count per annulus and the coefficient of variation were calculated for the eight reconstructions in fig. 3.24, over the entire reconstructed volume. As a control, data were synthesised that comprised a uniform cylinder with a uniform count distribution which had Poisson noise added that was equivalent to the noise level measured on each plane in a large region of interest on the final image in fig. 3.24d, *i.e.*, the most uniform image. The data are shown in fig. 3.28.

The nonuniformity index in this control is totally attributable to random statistical fluctuations alone, and therefore provides a comparison at the same count level as in the reconstructed sections of the "best case" results. In the non scatter corrected data, the nonuniformity index of the mean count is reasonably constant for each of the different corrections. This suggests that another factor is dominating this figure and the reconstructed images would suggest that it is the scatter. The variability in the mean count from centre to the edge of the cylinder dominates this measure. The lowest nonuniformity measure for the non scatter corrected data is in fig. 3.23b where the "scatter build-up" effectively offsets the hole caused by not correcting for the geometric profile. The radial coefficient of variation nonuniformity index decreases markedly with detector efficiency correction but changes little after that.

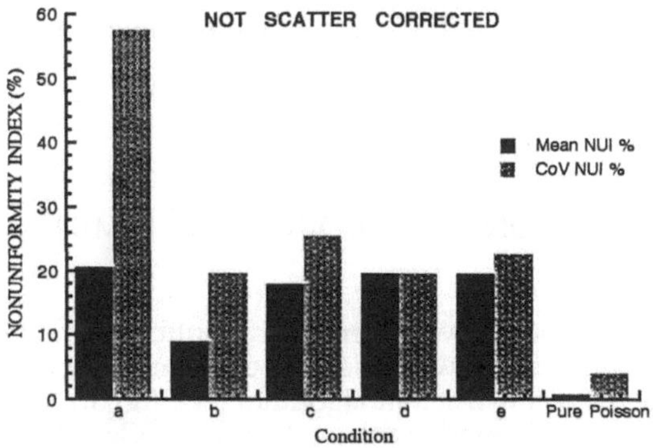

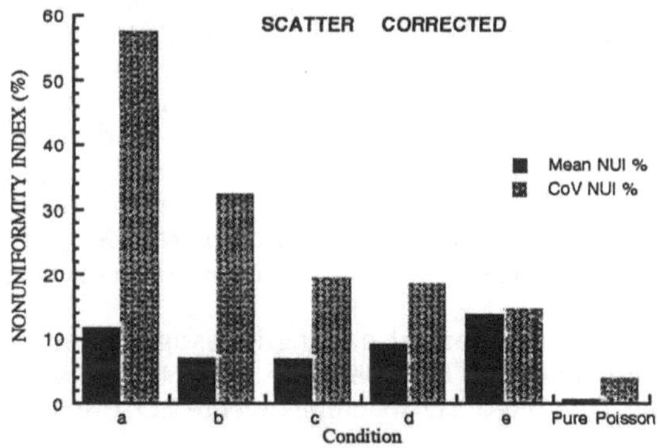

Figure 3.28. The graph on the top shows the nonuniformity index for all of the studies without scatter correction with successive columns demonstrating the effect of each extra correction. The graph on the bottom shows the same for the scatter corrected data. The corrections indicated match the image legends in fig. 3.23 and indicate condition 'a' (no normalisation), 'b' (detector efficiency only), 'c' (detector efficiency plus geometric profile), 'd' (detector efficiency plus geometric profile plus crystal interference) and 'e' (direct normalisation). The darker bars show the nonuniformity index value for the mean counts, while the lighter shaded bars show the nonuniformity index for the coefficient of variation between rings.

Again, the scatter appears to mask the underlying effects. The scatter corrected data firstly demonstrates that the mean count nonuniformity index is lower as there is little difference between the centre and edges of the cylinder (see fig. 3.25). Due to this, the mean count nonuniformity index now reflects the noise in the reconstructions, rather than the systematic error caused by the scatter build-up towards the centre of the object. The mean count nonuniformity index is seen to be highest for the data which used the direct normalisation, and probably reflects the noise propagated from the normalisation data. For these data with approximately $\sim 10^3$ counts per pixel, the statistical noise level in the sinogram for any individual detector was found to be ~15%-20%, rather than the naïve estimate of ~3% that would be expected from Poisson statistics. The coefficient of variation nonuniformity measure in the scatter corrected data is dominated by the geometric patterns, and as each extra correction is incorporated within the indirect approaches it is seen to decrease further. The direct normalisation displays the lowest value reflecting the fact that almost all of the geometric factors have been removed, apart from the remaining artefact in the centre of the scanner.

Attenuation Correction for 3D PET

ATTENUATION CORRECTION WITH COINCIDENCE MEASUREMENTS IN 3D PET

Attenuation correction has been given even less attention than normalisation for 3D PET. The original implementation which is still commonly used is analogous to the reprojection step in the 3D reconstruction algorithm (see fig. 3.1): the transmission and blank data are measured in 2D mode with septa using ^{68}Ge rotating rod sources from which the $\log_e$ transformed blank-to-transmission ratio images are reconstructed. A full set of 3D "attenuation" data are then formed by forward projection of this volume to give correction factors for each line-of-response in the measured 3D emission dataset [Townsend et al., 1989; McKee et al., 1991]. This is essentially a practical issue as most 2D/3D scanners are used in both 2D and 3D modes, and the transmission source strengths are usually chosen as those appropriate for 2D acquisition mode. The detectors would have impractically high deadtime if the septa were removed and these sources were used in 3D mode. In addition, the scatter fraction in the transmission data would be high, leading to underestimation of the attenuation coefficients.

Alternative acquisition geometries are also being investigated, such as an uncollimated flood or plane positron sources [Townsend et al., 1993; McKee and Hiltz, 1994; Townsend et al., 1994a] for fixed 3D machines where 2D transmission measurements are not an option.

SINGLE PHOTON APPROACHES FOR ATTENUATION CORRECTION

Full 3D transmission measurements using single photons rather than annihilation coincidence counting, as suggested initially by Derenzo with ^{133}Ba [Derenzo et al., 1975], are starting to appear, firstly using single photon measurements from a positron emitter [deKemp and Nahmias, 1994], and more recently using a pure single photon emitting source [Karp et al., 1995; Yu and Nahmias, 1995]. ^{137}Cs is attractive because of its long half life (30.1 years), almost appropriate energy (662 keV), relative abundance and hence low cost. The recently developed fully 3D tomograph "EXACT3D", installed at the MRC Cyclotron Unit, Hammersmith Hospital, which is the first full ring fixed 3D whole body tomograph [Jones et al., 1996], uses a point source of ~150 MBq of ^{137}Cs in a fluid drive to measure single photon flux for transmission [Jones et al., 1995]. There are two implications of using a ^{137}Cs point source for transmission measurements: the attenuation factors measured require scaling from the higher energy of the ^{137}Cs gamma photons to the 0.511 MeV annihilation coincidence photon energy of the emission source, and these measurements will have a large proportion of scattered photons, as this is essentially an "uncollimated" system. Point source single photon measurements appear to be the most promising method for transmission scanning in fully 3D tomographs and are discussed below.

Processing of Single Photon Data from 3D Measurements. Transmission data that rely on the detection of photons in singles rather than coincidence mode no longer restrict the choice of transmission sources to those that decay by positron emission. However, transmission data obtained using photons with energies other than 0.511 MeV must be extrapolated to give values as if they had been measured with 0.511 MeV photons. Attenuation correction factors, the ratio of the blank (I_0) to the transmission (I) scans, measured at one energy can be extrapolated to those that would have been measured at another energy using:

$$\left[\frac{I_0}{I}\right]_{0.511} = \left[\frac{I_0}{I}\right]_{EF} \qquad [3.15]$$

where F is the ratio of the mass attenuation coefficient for water at 0.511 MeV to that at E MeV [Yu et al., 1995].

As scattered events are acquired inevitably along with unscattered events, some processing of the transmission data are essential in order not to underestimate the measured attenuation coefficients [Digby and Hoffman, 1989]. Scatter correction can be applied on-the-fly during dual energy acquisition by choosing two non-overlapping windows such that the ratio of the scattered events in the photopeak window to the sum of the unscattered and scattered events in the lower scatter window is equal to unity [Grootoonk et al., 1991; Yu et al., 1995].

Statistical noise in the transmission measurements can increase significantly the noise level in the reconstructed emission images [Huang et al., 1979]. Smoothing of the transmission sinograms has been suggested to reduce statistical fluctuations [Dahlbom and Hoffman, 1987]. A different approach has been to segment the transmission images into a number of discrete regions, to assign appropriate linear attenuation coefficients to each of these regions, and to calculate attenuation correction factors using these noiseless estimates. Transmission images can be segmented manually by having an operator draw the various regions of interest [Huang et al., 1981], or automatically by applying thresholds to the pixel intensity histogram [Xu et al., 1991; Xu et al., 1994]. Discrete values for the attenuation coefficients have then been assumed to be the average of the reconstructed attenuation coefficient in each of these segmented regions. Meikle [Meikle et al., 1993] used the pixel intensity histogram of a transmission image to estimate the probabilities of a pixel belonging to one of three tissue types: air, lung or soft tissue. The appropriate linear attenuation coefficient to be assigned to each pixel is then calculated as the sum of the product of the estimated probabilities and the corresponding theoretical attenuation coefficient for each of the three tissue types. Xu's method uses a local area thresholding technique to allow for regional variability within an organ [Xu et al., 1994], which is particularly important in the lungs where the pooling of blood causes anterior-posterior and apical-basal gradations in the gross lung density.

A different approach that uses artificial neural networks (ANN) has recently been introduced [Yu and Nahmias, 1996]. This approach allows for the incorporation of local neighbourhood data in the classification of pixels, making the method less susceptible to noise. The outputs from the ANN are the conditional probabilities of each pixel belonging to one of three classes. The introduction and validation of a calibration curve, relating one of these conditional probabilities to absolute values of linear attenuation coefficients, removes the requirement for scatter correction of the transmission data. Furthermore, this approach allows for the calculation of more precise attenuation correction factors as the method is sensitive to the local variations in attenuation coefficients that are expected in the clinical situation. This technique was shown to provide accurate, subject independent, and reproducible attenuation data without the need for scatter correction. It can predict accurately the value of the attenuation coefficient for any material in the range from air to water [Yu et al., 1996].

In practice, accurate attenuation correction factors can be obtained by acquiring a short transmission scan using the singles transmission measurement technique, and then processing these data using a knowledge based approach, such as the one that uses artificial neural networks. This, and other processing methods which use *a priori* knowledge, offer great promise for producing high quality transmission scans, especially in the post-injection mode, which is critical for producing accurate, quantitative reconstructed data in the clinic.

Calibration in 3D PET

For 3D PET to be accepted as being a quantitative biochemical tool in the way that 2D PET is, accurate calibration of the reconstructed images in units of activity per unit volume (or *quantification*) is required. This implies accurate corrections for physical and instrumental factors such as photon attenuation and scatter, correcting for differences in detector efficiencies and geometric normalisation, as well as having a suitable method for calibrating the device. Calibration allows the reconstructed image concentrations to be related to other measures of the radioactivity related to the study, *e.g.*, the percentage of the dose administered that is taken up by the target tissue, the concentration of the tracer in the blood and tissue at some point in time, *etc.* Two basic approaches exist: relative (cross) calibration and absolute calibration.

CROSS-CALIBRATION

In 2D PET the usual method for calibrating the reconstructed data is by *cross-calibration* of a water-filled cylinder against a well-counter [Eichling et al., 1977]. A suitable radionuclide of a known concentration of radioactivity is uniformly distributed in the cylinder. Scatter correction in 2D PET is often ignored because of the low scatter fraction. Furthermore, it is assumed in 2D PET that the scatter from the cylinder will be of approximately the same order as it will in the head, thorax, or abdomen in a human study providing further justification for ignoring it. In 3D PET, however, due to the high scatter fraction in such an object, the uniform cylinder used for calibration will require scatter correction. Thus, with a cross calibration approach *the accuracy of the calibration is dependent on the efficacy of the scatter correction of the calibration object,* and further, on the accuracy of the scatter correction for different regions of the body where the correction required will vary greatly (head *c.f.* thorax *c.f.* abdomen). This is less of an issue in 2D PET as the fraction of scattered events is much less. One investigator who has questioned the validity of cross-calibration with a 20 cm diameter cylinder for 3D PET is Cherry [Cherry et al., 1993], who calibrated his system from the reconstructed image of a 3 cm diameter by 3 cm long cylinder with a calculated attenuation correction, assuming that the scatter from such an object would be sufficiently small as to be ignored. This method is a cross-calibration approach that does not require scatter correction (or, more accurately, for one in which scatter is not a major contribution). One criticism of this method is that the object only occupies a small portion of the axial field of view. The axial response profile in a reconstructed volume is susceptible to significant variations, and it may be necessary to measure the calibration at different axial locations.

ABSOLUTE CALIBRATION

To date, most papers dealing with scatter correction of 3D PET data have only compared *relative* concentrations within different regions of the same test object, with one section serving as a reference region [Shao et al., 1991; Bailey et al., 1994; Lercher et al., 1994; Shao et al., 1994]. Clearly, this does not reflect the *accuracy* of the correction technique. Absolute calibration is the direct measurement of the sensitivity of the scanner, ideally without corrections for scatter, attenuation, *etc.* This is easily achieved in SPECT, for example, where a calibrated amount of a single photon emitting radionuclide can be measured and the count rate in air determined under conditions of minimal attenuation and scattering. However, in PET, as the positron requires a finite amount of surrounding media in which to annihilate, and because this amount of material will attenuate some of the photons, a simple calibration "in air" is not possible. One approach that has attempted to overcome this limitation was the extension of a method previously developed to measure the sensitivity of an emission tomographic device in units of counts per second per unit radioactivity [Bailey et al., 1991]. The technique uses multiple measurements of a source with increasing attenuation of the source which does not require scatter or attenuation correction and therefore gives a calibration independent of the effects of scatter and attenuation [Bailey and Jones, 1997]. For calibrating reconstructed images, though, it is performed on reconstructed data and therefore undergoes the same normalisation and reconstruction steps (*i.e.*, filtering, zoom, interpolation) as do clinical studies. The motivation for the development of this method was primarily to obtain an independent calibration with which to assess various scatter correction techniques. The method allows the user to calculated the concentration in the object by using the simple relation

$$A(\text{kBq.pixel}^{-1}) = \frac{f_R(\text{ct.s}^{-1}\text{.pixel}^{-1}\text{.plane}^{-1})}{C(\text{ct.s}^{-1}\text{.plane}^{-1}\text{.kBq}^{-1})} \qquad [3.16]$$

where f_R is the reconstructed count rate per pixel and C is the factor determined from the absolute calibration.

Acknowledgement

The extensive assistance of Dr Claude Comtat in the preparation of this Chapter is gratefully acknowledged.

References

Axelsson B, Msaki P, and Israelsson A (1984): "Subtraction of Compton-scattered photons in single-photon emission computerized tomography" J Nucl Med 25: 490-494

Bailey DL, Hutton BF, Meikle SR, Fulton RR, and Jackson CB (1989a): "An attenuation dependent scatter correction technique for SPECT" Phys Med Biol 34: 152 (Abstract)

Bailey DL, Hutton BF, Meikle SR, Fulton RR, and Jackson CB (1989b): "Iterative scatter correction incorporating attenuation data" Eur J Nucl Med 15: 452 (Abstract)

Bailey DL and Jones T (1995): "Normalisation for 3D PET with a Translating Line

Pseudo-Plane Source" J Nucl Med 36(5): 92P (Abstract)

Bailey DL and Jones T (1997): "A method for calibrating three-dimensional positron emission tomography without scatter correction" Eur J Nucl Med 24(6): 660-664

Bailey DL, Jones T, and Spinks TJ (1991): "A Method for Measuring the Absolute Sensitivity of Positron Emission Tomographic Scanners" Eur J Nucl Med 18: 374-379

Bailey DL and Meikle SR (1994): "A convolution-subtraction scatter correction method for 3D PET" Phys Med Biol 39(3): 411-424

Bailey DL, Townsend DW, Kinahan PE, Grootoonk S, and Jones T (1996): "An Investigation of Factors Affecting Detector and Geometric Correction in Normalisation of 3D PET Data" IEEE Trans Nucl Sci NS-43: 1300-1307

Barney JS, Harrop R, and Dykstra CJ (1993): "Source Distribution Dependent Scatter Correction for PVI" IEEE Trans Nucl Sci NS-40(4): 1001-1007

Barney JS, Rogers J, Harrop R, and Hoverath H (1991): "Object shape dependent simulations for PET" IEEE Trans Nucl Sci NS-38(2): 719-725

Beck RN, Schuh MW, Cohen TD, and Lembares N (1969): "Effects of Scattered Radiation on Scintillation Detector Response". In: Medical Radioisotope Scintigraphy. Vienna: IAEA, Vol 1: pp. 595-615

Bendriem B, Trébossen R, Froulin V, and Syrota A (1993): "A PET Scatter Correction Using Simultaneous Acquisitions with Low and High Lower Energy Thresholds". In: Klaisner L, ed. Proceedings of the IEEE Nuclear Science Symposium and Medical Imaging Conference, San Francisco, USA. Vol 3:1779-1783

Bentourkia M, Msaki P, Cadorette J, and Lecomte R (1993): "Assessment of Scatter Components in Multispectral PET Imaging". In: Klaisner L, ed. Proceedings of the IEEE Nuclear Science Symposium and Medical Imaging Conference, San Francisco, USA. Vol 3:1505-1509

Bentourkia M, Msaki P, Cadorette J, and Lecomte R (1995): "Energy Dependence of Scatter Components in Multispectral PET Imaging" IEEE Trans Nucl Sci NS-14(1): 138-145

Bergström M, Eriksson L, Bohm C, Blomqvist G, and Litton J-E (1983): "Correction for scattered radiation in a ring detector positron camera by integral transformation of the projections" J Comput Assist Tomogr 7(1): 42-50

Bergström M, Eriksson L, Greitz T, Litton J, and Widen L (1982): "A Procedure for Calibrating and Correcting Data to Achieve Accurate Quantitative Values in Positron Emission Tomography" IEEE Trans Nucl Sci NS-29(1): 555-557

Casey ME, Gadagkar H, and Newport D (1995): "A Component Based Method for Normalization in Volume PET". In: Grangeat P and Amans J-L, eds. Proceedings of the 3rd International Conference on Three-Dimensional Image Reconstruction in Radiology and Nuclear Medicine, Aix-les-Bains. Vol 67-71

Casey ME and Hoffman EJ (1986): "Quantitation in positron emission tomography: 7. A technique to reduce noise in accidental coincidence measurement and coincidence efficiency calibration" J Comput Assist Tomogr 10(5): 845-850

Cherry SR, Dahlbom M, and Hoffman EJ (1991): "3D PET using a Conventional Multislice Tomograph without Septa" J Comput Assist Tomogr 15: 655-668

Cherry SR, Dahlbom M, and Hoffman EJ (1992): "Evaluation of a 3D reconstruction algorithm for multi-slice PET scanners" Phys Med Biol 37: 779-790

Cherry SR and Huang S-C (1995): "Effects of Scatter on Model Parameter Estimates in 3D PET Studies of the Human Brain" IEEE Trans Nucl Sci NS-42(4): 1174-1179

Cherry SR, Meikle SR, and Hoffman EJ (1993): "Correction and Characterization of Scattered Events in Three-Dimensional PET Using Scanners with Retractable Septa" J Nucl Med 34: 671-678

Chesler DA and Stearns CW (1990): "Calibration of detector sensitivity in positron cameras" IEEE Trans Nucl Sci 37(2): 768-772

Compton AH (1923): "A quantum theory of the scattering of X-rays by light elements" Phys Rev 21: 483-502

Dahlbom M and Hoffman EJ (1987): "Problems in signal-to-noise ratio for attenuation correction in high resolution PET" IEEE Trans Nucl Sci 34(1): 288-293

Defrise M, Townsend DW, Bailey DL, Geissbühler A, Michel C, and Jones T (1991): "A normalization technique for 3D PET data" Phys Med Biol 36(7): 939-952

deKemp RA and Nahmias C (1994): "Attenuation correction in PET using single photon transmission measurement" Med Phys 21(6): 771-778

Derenzo SE, Zaklad H, and Budinger TF (1975): "Analytical study of a high-resolution positron ring detector system for transaxial reconstruction tomography" J Nucl Med 16(12): 1166-1173

DeVito R, Hamill J, Trefert J, and Stoub E (1989): "Energy-weighted acquisition of scintigraphic images by analysis of energy spectra" J Nucl Med 30: 2029-2035

Digby WM and Hoffman EJ (1989): "An investigation of scatter in attenuation correction for PET" IEEE Trans Nucl Sci NS-36(1): 1038-1042

Egbert SD and May RS (1980): "An integral-transport method for Compton-scatter correction in emission computed tomography" IEEE Trans Nucl Sci NS-27(1): 543-547

Eichling JO, Higgins CS, and Ter-Pogossian MM (1977): "Determination of Radionuclide Concentrations with Positron CT Scanning (PETT): Concise Communication" J Nucl Med 18: 845-847

Erhardt JC, Oberley LW, and Lensink SC (1974): "Effect of Scattering Medium on Gamma-Ray Imaging" J Nucl Med 15: 934-938

Floyd CE, Jaszczak RT, Greer KL, and Coleman RE (1985): "Deconvolution of Compton scatter in SPECT" J Nucl Med 26: 403-408

Gagnon D, Todd-Pokropek A, Arsenault A, and Dupras G (1989): "Introduction to holospectral imaging in nuclear medicine for scatter subtraction" IEEE Trans Med Imag MI-8: 245-250

Goggin AS and Ollinger JM (1994): "A model for multiple scatters in fully 3D PET". In: Trendler RC, ed. Proceedings of the IEEE Nuclear Science Symposium and Medical Imaging Conference, Norfolk, VA, USA. Vol 4:1609-1613

Grootoonk S, Spinks TJ, Jones T, Michel C, and Bol A (1991): "Correction for scatter using a dual energy window technique with a tomograph operated without septa". In: Proceedings of the IEEE Nuclear Science Symposium and Medical Imaging Conference, Santa Fe. Vol 3:1569-1573

Harrison RL, Haynor DR, and Lewellen TK (1991): "Dual energy window scatter corrections for PET". In: Proceedings of the IEEE Nuclear Science Symposium and Medical Imaging Conference, Santa Fe. Vol 3:1700-1704

Haynor DR, Kaplan MS, Miyaoka RS, and Lewellen TK (1995): "Multi-window scatter correction techniques in single-photon imaging" Med Phys 22(12): 2015-2024

Hiltz LG and McKee BTA (1994): "Scatter correction for three-dimensional PET based on an analytical model dependent on source and attenuating object" Phys Med Biol 39: 2059-2071

Hoffman EJ, Guerrero TM, Germano G, Digby WM, and Dahlbom M (1989): "PET system calibration and corrections for quantitative and spatially accurate imagees" IEEE Trans Nucl Sci 36(1): 1108-1112

Huang S-C, Carson R, Phelps ME, Hoffman EJ, Schelbert H, and Kuhl D (1981): "A boundary method for attenuation correction in positron emission tomography" IEEE Trans Nucl Sci 22: 627–637

Huang SC, Hoffman EJ, Phelps ME, and Kuhl DE (1979): "Quantitation in positron emission tomography: 2. Effect of inaccurate attenuation correction" J Comput Assist Tomogr 3(6): 804-814

Jaszczak RJ, Greer KL, Floyd CE, Harris CG, and Coleman RE (1984): "Improved SPECT quantitation using compensation for scattered photons" J Nucl Med 25: 893-900

Jones T, Bailey DL, Bloomfield PM, et al (1996): "Performance Characteristics And Novel Design Aspects Of The Most Sensitive PET Camera Built For High Temporal And Spatial Resolution" J Nucl Med 37(5): 85P(Abstract)

Jones WF, Vaigneur K, Young J, Moyers C, and Nahmias C (1995): "The Architectural Impact of Single Photon Transmission Measurements on Full Ring 3D Positron Tomography". In: Moonier PA, ed. Proceedings of the IEEE Nuclear Science Symposium and Medical Imaging Conference, San Francisco. Vol 2:1026-1030

Karp JS, Daube-Witherspoon ME, Hoffman EJ, et al (1991): "Performance Standards in Positron Emission Tomography" J Nucl Med 32(12): 2342-2350

Karp JS, Muehllehner G, Qu H, and Yan X-H (1995): "Singles transmission in volume-imaging PET with a ^{137}Cs source" Phys Med Biol 40: 929-944

Karp JS, Muehllener G, Mankoff DA, Ordonez CE, Ollinger JM, Daube-Witherspoon ME, Haigh AT, and Beerbohm DJ (1990): "Continuous-slice PENN-PET: a positron tomograph with volume imaging capability" J Nucl Med 31: 617-627

Kinahan PE and Rogers JG (1989): "Analytic 3-D image reconstruction using all detected events" IEEE Trans Nucl Sci NS-36: 964-968

Kinahan PE, Townsend DW, Bailey DL, Sashin D, Jadali F, and Mintun MA (1995): "Efficiency Normalization Techniques for 3D PET Data". In: Moonier PA, ed. Proceedings of the IEEE Nuclear Science Symposium and Medical Imaging Conference, San Francisco. Vol 2:1021-1025

King M, Schwinger R, Doherty P, and Penney B (1984): "Two-dimensional filtering of SPECT images using the Metz and Weiner filters" J Nucl Med 25: 1234-1240

King MA, Hademenos GJ, and Glick SJ (1992): "A dual-photopeak window method for scatter correction" J Nucl Med 33: 605-612

Klein O and Nishina Y (1928): "Uber die streuung von strahlung durch frei elektronen nach der neuen relativistischen quantendynamik von Dirac" Z Physik 52: 853-868

Koral KF, Clinthorne NH, and Rogers WL (1986): "Improving emission-computed-tomography quantification by compton-scatter rejection through offset windows" Nucl Instr Meth Phys Res A242: 610-614

Larsson SA (1980): "Gamma camera emission tomography. Development and properties of a multi-sectional emission computed tomography system" Acta Radiol Suppl 363: 30-32

Lercher MJ and Wienhard K (1994): "Scatter Correction in 3-D PET" IEEE Trans Med Imag MI-13(4): 649-657

Levin CS, Dahlbom M, and Hoffman EJ (1995): "A Monte Carlo Correction for the Effect of Compton Scattering in 3-D PET Brain Imaging" IEEE Trans Nucl Sci NS-42(4): 1181-1185

Links JM, Leal JP, Mueller-Gartner HW, and Wagner Jr HN (1992): "Improved positron emission tomography quantification by Foruier-based restoration filtering" Eur J Nucl Med 19: 925-932

Ljungberg M and Strand S-E (1990): "Scatter and attenuation correction in SPECT using density maps and Monte Carlo simulated scatter functions" J Nucl Med 31: 1560-1567

McKee B, Clack R, Harvey P, Hiltz L, Hogan M, and Howse D (1991): "Accurate attenuation correction for a 3D PET system" Phys Med Biol 36(5): 603-619

McKee BTA, Gurvey AT, Harvey PJ, and Howse DC (1992): "A Deconvolution Scatter Correction for a 3-D PET System" IEEE Trans Med Imag MI-11(4): 560-569

McKee BTA and Hiltz LG (1994): "Attenuation correction for three-dimensional PET using uncollimated flood-source transmission measurements" Phys Med Biol 39: 2043-2058

Meikle SR, Dahlbom M, and Cherry SR (1993): "Attenuation correction using count-limited transmission data in positron emission tomography" J Nucl Med 34(1): 143-150

Meikle SR, Hutton BF, and Bailey DL (1994): "A transmission dependent method for scatter correction in SPECT" J Nucl Med 35(2): 360-367

Meikle SR, Hutton BF, Bailey DL, Fulton RR, and Schindhelm K (1991): "SPECT scatter correction in non-homogeneous media". In: Colchester ACF and Hawkes DJ, Information Processing in Medical Imaging: XIIth IPMI International Conference. Berlin: Springer-Verlag, pp. 34-44

Msaki P, Axelsson B, Dahl CM, and Larsson SA (1987): "Generalized scatter correction method in SPECT using point scatter distribution functions" J Nucl Med 28: 1861-1869

Mumcuoglu EU, Leahy R, Cherry SR, and Zhou Z (1994): "Fast Gradient Based Methods for Bayesian Reconstruction of Transmission and Emission PET Images" IEEE Trans Med Imag MI-13: 687-701

Naude H, van Aswegen A, Herbst CP, Lotter MG, and Pretorius PH (1996): "A Monte Carlo evaluation of the channel ratio scatter correction method" Phys Med Biol 41: 1059-1066

NEMA (1986): Performance measurements of scintillation cameras. Standards Publication NU-1-1986, National Electrical Manufacturers Association, Washington, DC

Ollinger J (1991): "Estimation of the distribution of scattered coincidences in PET using transmission scans" J Nucl Med 32: 996

Ollinger JM (1995): "Detector Efficiency and Compton Scatter in Fully 3D PET" IEEE Trans Nucl Sci NS-42(4): 1168-1173

Ollinger JM (1996): "Model-based scatter correction for fully 3D PET" Phys Med Biol 41(1): 153-176

Ollinger JM and Johns GC (1993): "Model-Based Scatter Correction for Fully 3D PET". In: Klaisner L, ed. Proceedings of the IEEE Nuclear Science Symposium and Medical Imaging Conference, San Francisco, USA. Vol 3:1264-1268

Penney BC, Rajeevan N, Bushe HS, Hademenos G, and King MA (1991): "A scatter reduction method for In-111 scintigrams using five energy windows". In: Baldwin GT, ed. Proceedings of the IEEE Nuclear Science Symposium and Medical Imaging Conference, Santa Fe. Vol 3:1866-1873

Prati P, Lanza P, Corveisiero P, Guzzardi R, and Sorace O (1993): "Verification of the integral transformation of the projection technique for scatter correction in positron tomographs" Eur J Nucl Med 20: 255-259

Pretorious P, van Rensburg A, van Aswegen A, Lötter M, Serfontein D, and Herbst C (1993): "The Channel Ratio method of Scatter Correction for Radionuclide Image Quantitation" J Nucl Med 34: 330-335

Rakshi J, Bailey DL, Morrish PK, and Brooks DJ (1996): "Implementation of 3D Acquisition, Reconstruction and Analysis of Dynamic Fluorodopa Studies". In: Myers R, Cunningham VJ, Bailey DL and Jones T, Quantification of Brain Function Using PET. San Diego: Academic Press, pp. 82-87

Shao L, Freifelder R, and Karp JS (1994): "Triple Energy Window Scatter Correction Technique in PET" IEEE Trans Med Imag 13(4): 641-648

Shao L and Karp JS (1991): "Cross-Plane Scattering Correction - Point Source Deconvolution in PET" IEEE Trans Med Imag MI-10(3): 234-239

Shao L and Karp JS (1995): "Modified Convolution-Subtraction Scattering Correction Technique for 3D PET". In: Proceedings of the IEEE Nuclear Science Symposium and Medical Imaging Conference, San Francisco. Vol (to appear)

Shao L, Karp JS, and Freifelder R (1993): "Composite dual window scattering correction technique in PET". In: Klaisner L, ed. Proceedings of the IEEE Nuclear Science Symposium and Medical Imaging Conference, San Francisco, USA. Vol 3:1391-1395

Spinks TJ, Jones T, Bailey DL, Townsend DW, Grootoonk S, Bloomfield PM, Gilardi M-C, Sipe B, and Reed J (1992): "Physical performance of a positron tomograph for brain imaging with retractable septa" Phys Med Biol 37(8): 1637-1655

Stazyk MW, Sossi V, Buckley KR, and Ruth TJ (1994): "Normalization Measurement in Septa-less PET Scanners" J Nucl Med 35(5): 41P (Abstract)

Stearns CW (1995): "Scatter Correction Methods for 3D PET Using 2D Fitted Gaussian Functions" J Nucl Med 36(5): 105P(Abstract)

Thompson CJ (1993): "The Problem of Scatter Correction in Positron Volume Imaging" IEEE Trans Med Imag MI-10: 234-239

Townsend DW, Bishop H, Mintun MA, Byars LG, Geissbühler A, and Nutt R (1994a): "Physical and Clinical Performance of a Rotating Positron Tomograph" J Nucl Med 35(5): 41P (Abstract)

Townsend DW, Choi Y, Sashin D, and Mintun M (1994b): "An Investigation of Practical Scatter Correction Techniques for 3D PET" J Nucl Med 35(5): 50P (Abstract)

Townsend DW, Geissbühler A, Defrise M, Hoffman EJ, Spinks TJ, Bailey DL, Gilardi M-C, and Jones T (1991): "Fully Three-Dimensional Reconstruction for a PET Camera with Retractable Septa" IEEE Trans Med Imag 10: 505-512

Townsend DW, Price JC, Mintun MA, Kinahan PE, Jadali F, Sashin D, Simpson N, and Mathis CA (1996): "Scatter Correction for Brain Receptor Quantitation in 3D PET". In: Myers R, Cunningham VJ, Bailey DL and Jones T, Quantification of Brain Function Using PET. San Diego: Academic Press, pp. 76-81

Townsend DW, Spinks TJ, Jones T, Geissbühler A, Defrise M, Gilardi M-C, and Heather JD (1989): "Three dimensional reconstruction of PET data from a multi-ring camera" IEEE Trans Nucl Sci 36(1): 1056-1065

Townsend DW, Wensveen M, Byars LG, Geissbühler A, Tochon-Danguy HJ, Christin A, Defrise M, Bailey DL, Grootoonk S, Donath A, and Nutt R (1993): "A Rotating PET Scanner Using BGO Block Detectors: Design, Performance and Applications" J Nucl Med 34: 1367-1376

Trébossen R and Bendriem B (1995a): "Quantitation in 3D PET; the effect of scatter correction on recovery coefficient". In: Grangeat P, ed. Proceedings of the 3rd International Meeting on Fully Three-Dimensional Image Reconstruction in Radiology and Nuclear Medicine, Aix-les-Bains, France. Vol 127-131

Trébossen R, Bendriem B, Fontaine A, Frouin V, and Remy P (1996): "Quantitation of the [18F]Fluorodopa Uptake in the Human Striatum in 3D PET with the ETM Scatter Correction". In: Myers R, Cunningham VJ, Bailey DL and Jones T, Quantification of Brain Function Using PET. San Diego: Academic Press, pp. 88-92

Trébossen R, Bendriem B, Fontaine A, Rougetet R, Frouin V, and Remy P (1995b): "Quantitation of Clinical 3D PET Studies with the ETM Scatter Correction". In: Moonier PA, ed. Proceedings of the IEEE Nuclear Science Symposium and Medical Imaging Conference, San Francisco. Vol 3:1447-1452

Watson CC, Newport D, and Casey ME (1996): "A Single Scatter Simulation Technique for Scatter Correction in 3D PET". In: Grangeat P and Amans J-L, Three-Dimensional Image Reconstruction in Radiology and Nuclear Medicine. Dordrecht: Kluwer Academic, (Viergever MA, ed. Computational Imaging and Vision; Vol 4: pp. 255-268

Wu C, Ordenez CE, and Chen C-T (1994): "Characterization and Correction for Scatter in 3D PET Using Rebinned Plane Integrals" IEEE Trans Nucl Sci NS-41(6): 2758-2764

Wu C, Ordonez CE, and Chen C-T (1993): "Scatter Correction for 3-D PET by Convolution of Plane-Integral Projections". In: Klaisner L, ed. Proceedings of the IEEE Nuclear Science Symposium and Medical Imaging Conference, San Francisco, USA. Vol 3:1515-1519

Xu EZ, Mullani NA, Gould KL, and Anderson WL (1991): "A segmented attenuation correction for PET" J Nucl Med 32: 161-165

Xu M, Luk WK, Cutler PD, and Digby WM (1994): "Local threshold for segmented attenuation correction of PET imaging of the thorax" IEEE Trans Nucl Sci NS-41: 1532-1537

Yanch JC, Flower MA, and Webb S (1990): "Improved quantification of radionuclide uptake using deconvolution and windowed subtraction techniques for scatter compensation in single photon emission computed tomography" Med Phys 17(6): 1011-1022

Yu SK and Nahmias C (1995): "Single-photon transmission measurements in positron emission tomography using ^{137}Cs" Phys Med Biol 40: 1255-1266

Yu SK and Nahmias C (1996): "Segmented attenuation correction using artificial neural networks in positron tomography" Phys Med Biol 41: 2189-2206

Chapter 4. VOLUME IMAGING TOMOGRAPHS

David W. Townsend[1], Roberto A. Isoardi[1,2]
and Bernard Bendriem[3]

[1] PET Facility, Department of Radiology, University of Pittsburgh, USA
[2] Fundacion Escuela de Medicina Nuclear, Mendoza, Argentina
[3] Service Hospitalier Frédéric Joliot, CEA, Orsay, France

Introduction

Although initially volume imaging scanners for PET were based on alternative technologies such as multiwire chambers [Townsend et al., 1987] and rotating dual head gamma cameras [Muehllehner, 1975], a significant advance occurred in 1990 with the appearance of the first commercial *multi-ring* PET scanner with volume imaging capability. This scanner, the ECAT 953B (CTI PET Systems, Knoxville, TN) [Mazoyer et al., 1991; Spinks et al., 1992] offered both 2D and 3D data acquisition by extending (2D) or retracting (3D) the septa, a procedure that took less than two minutes. The ECAT 953B provided, for the first time, a platform on which to compare 2D and 3D acquisition and to develop 3D methodology. Following the lead of CTI PET Systems (CPS), since 1991 all multi-ring PET scanners are now manufactured either with retractable septa, or are fully 3D and have no septa. The aim of this chapter is to review current tomograph hardware designs for 3D PET imaging, and to compare the 2D and 3D performance characteristics of the different commercially-available multi-ring scanners.

	ECAT 953B	ECAT EXACT	EXACT HR+	ADVANCE
Detector size (mm)	5.6 x 6.1 x 30	6.4 x 6.4 x 20	4.0 x 4.1 x 30	4.0 x 8.1 x 30
No. of detectors	6,144	9,216	18,432	12,096
No. of rings	16	24	32	18
No. of slices	31	47	63	35
Slice width (mm)	3.4	3.4	2.4	4.3
Ring diameter (cm)	76.0	82.4	82.7	92.7
Axial FOV (cm)	10.4	16.2	15.2	15.2
Max. axial angle	7.5°	10.7°	10.2°	8.8°

Table 4.1 Design specifications of multi-ring PET scanners with retractable septa

B. Bendriem and D.W. Townsend (eds.) The Theory and Practice of 3D PET, 111-132.

The design characteristics of some PET scanners with retractable septa are presented in table 4.1. The ECAT 953B had a 35 cm diameter patient port which essentially limited applications to the brain. This tomograph was followed by the whole body design, the ECAT 951R also with a 10.4 cm axial field-of-view (FOV), and by the ECAT EXACT [Wienhard et al., 1992] with an axial FOV increased to 16.2 cm. The next generation of scanners included the EXACT HR [Wienhard et al., 1994] and EXACT HR+ [Brix et al., 1997] manufactured by CPS, and the ADVANCE [DeGrado et al., 1994; Lewellen et al., 1995; Lewellen et al., 1996] from General Electric Medical Systems (GEMS, Milwaukee, WI), all with improved spatial resolution and a 15 cm axial FOV.

The design of two lower cost, fully 3D, PET scanners, the ECAT ART [Bailey et al., 1997] and the QUEST also take advantage of the increased sensitivity of 3D. In the ECAT ART, cost saving is achieved by reducing the number of detectors compared to a full ring design; dual arrays of detectors are rotated to acquire a full data set, and 3D acquisition ensures an adequate sensitivity even with the reduced number of detectors. The QUEST, built by UGM Medical Systems (Philadelphia, PA) and currently marketed by GEMS, comprises six large sodium iodide detectors in an hexagonal configuration. Cost saving is achieved by the use of sodium iodide (NaI), a less expensive detector material than bismuth germanate (BGO) used in the ECAT and ADVANCE scanners, and by the smaller number of photomultiplier tubes required. Acquisition in 3D offsets the lower intrinsic sensitivity of sodium iodide compared to BGO at 511 keV, ensuring an adequate sensitivity. Finally, the successful development of 3D methodology led recently to the appearance of the first commercial, multi-ring scanner without septa, the EXACT3D [Jones et al., 1996; Spinks et al., 1997] from CPS. The EXACT3D comprises 27,648 detectors and covers an axial extent of 23.4 cm. Some design characteristics of these fully 3D PET scanners are shown in table 4.2.

	ECAT ART	QUEST	EXACT3D
Detector size (mm)	6.4 x 6.4 x 20	500 x 300 x 25	4.1 x 4.4 x 30
No. of detectors	6,144	6	27,648
No. of rings	24	*	48
No. of slices	47	128	95
Slice width (mm)	3.4	1.9	2.4
Ring diameter (cm)	82	85	82
Axial FOV (cm)	16.2	25	23.4
Max. axial angle	11.3°	16.4°	16.2°

Table 4.2 Design specifications of fully 3D PET scanners
* The QUEST has continuous sampling and is not a multi-ring device

Performance Characteristics

The physical performance characteristics of PET tomographs can be specified in terms of parameters such as in-plane and axial spatial resolution, sensitivity, count rate capability and deadtime, scatter fraction and image uniformity. Measurements are made with phantoms such as line sources and 20 cm diameter uniform cylinders according to standards defined by the National Electrical Manufacturers Association

(NEMA) protocols [Karp et al., 1991]. These measurements reflect the performance of the scanner and provide a basis on which to compare different tomographs. However, it is difficult to realistically evaluate overall scanner performance based on comparisons of a single parameter such as spatial resolution or maximum count rate. A similar situation arises in the comparison of the 2D and 3D performance of a given scanner. While retracting the septa obviously results in an increase in true counts, there is a corresponding increase in scatter and randoms, and there may also be a degradation in spatial resolution. The noise equivalent count rate (NEC) concept [Strother et al., 1987] was proposed to account for the different true, randoms and scatter rates that arise between different tomographs with a given activity distribution in the field of view. This concept has also proved useful to compare the 2D vs 3D count rate performance of different tomographs [Bailey at al., 1991a].

In the following sections, the physical performance parameters are discussed in relation to differences between 2D and 3D PET methodology. Comparative measurements are given for a number of different PET scanners. All values are summarized at the end of the section in table 4.3 for scanners with retractable septa, and table 4.4 for fully 3D, septaless scanners.

SPATIAL RESOLUTION

Transaxial, or in-plane, spatial resolution is measured according to the NEMA protocol by imaging a line source of activity in air aligned parallel with the axis of the scanner at different locations within the FOV, such as centred, and at radii of 4 cm and 8 cm. The line source data are reconstructed in 2D with a ramp filter with no smoothing, and in 3D with a Colsher filter [Colsher, 1980] with no smoothing (equivalent to the ramp filter in 2D), and the full width half maximum (FWHM) estimated for a profile through the source. The factors which limit tomograph resolution include the physical effects of positron range and photon acollinearity (see Chapter 1), the detector size, and an effect due to the block-based design of current tomographs [Derenzo et al., 1993]. Even though the profile is usually specified by the FWHM, the characteristics of the entire profile (termed the line, or point, spread function) are of interest, particularly since the tails of the function may differ significantly from those of a Gaussian distribution.

In 2D, the septa cover a small fraction of the crystal length, reducing the apparent crystal size in the axial direction. In most tomographs, only small differences in transaxial (in-plane) spatial resolution are observed between measurements in 2D and 3D for the central axial planes (table 4.3). The resolution is observed to degrade towards the edge of the axial FOV, due to the smoothing effect of the reprojection step in the reconstruction algorithm (Chapter 2) which contributes more synthetic data to the axial extremities than to the centre. For the HR+, at a radius of 1 cm, the mean resolution averaged over the central thirty planes is 4.5 mm x 4.7 mm (tangential x radial), compared to 5.1 mm x 4.9 mm averaged over all axial planes. For a scanner with circular geometry, at transaxial locations away from the centre of the tomograph, a degradation of the radial component of resolution is observed in both 2D and 3D. This degradation is caused by the increasingly-oblique incidence of photons on the front face of the detectors with increasing distance from the centre of the tomograph. In future tomograph designs, the availability of depth-of-interaction information will improve spatial resolution away from the centre of the FOV. Measurements of transaxial resolution in a scattering medium (uniform cylinder of water) show a slight degradation (< 0.5 mm), a little more in 3D than 2D.

In 2D, axial resolution is measured by stepping a point source in small increments (0.5 mm) through the FOV in the axial direction and noting the count rate at each position, a measurement that is related to axial slice width rather than to resolution. In 3D, the axial resolution is again measured by stepping a point source in small increments, but in this case the data are collected and reconstructed. The FWHM of a profile along the axial direction through the reconstructed point source yields an estimate of axial resolution. Stepping the source allows the variation of the measured resolution with axial position to be determined. For the HR+ scanner, similar values are measured for axial resolution in both 2D and 3D (table 4.3), and for a given transaxial position, the values show little axial variation throughout the FOV. Slight degradation of the axial resolution is also observed in a scattering medium, a little more in 3D than 2D.

A somewhat less favourable situation arises with the ADVANCE owing to the use of rectangular crystals in the tomograph (see table 4.1). In the transaxial direction, the crystals have the same dimension as those in the HR+ (4 mm), and thus a similar resolution is measured in 2D and 3D for both tomographs. However, in the axial direction, the crystals in the ADVANCE are twice the dimension of the crystals in the HR+. With the septa in place, an axial resolution of 4-4.5 mm is measured for both the ADVANCE and the HR+, whereas the axial resolution at the centre of the FOV in 3D is 6 mm for the ADVANCE and 4 mm for the HR+. This degradation of axial resolution in 3D in the ADVANCE is a consequence of the 8.1 mm axial dimension of the crystals compared with 4.1 mm in the HR+. The loss of axial resolution in the ADVANCE may be important when imaging small structures in the brain in 3D. To ensure isotropic resolution in 3D, crystals of square cross-section (uniform sampling) are to be preferred.

SENSITIVITY

The single most important advantage of 3D PET is the increase in sensitivity due to the increase in the effective geometrical solid angle covered by the tomograph when the septa are retracted. It is usual to characterize the change in sensitivity from 2D to 3D by measuring the volume sensitivity of a standard phantom, a 20 cm diameter uniform cylinder. The measurement of volume sensitivity according to the NEMA protocol is based on the count rate obtained with the cylinder containing a low radioactivity concentration of around 3.7 kBq/ml (0.1 μCi/ml). A low activity concentration is chosen to minimise the effects of deadtime and randoms (< 1%), so as to provide an accurate measure of the scanner sensitivity. The true activity concentration is obtained by taking aliquots of activity from the phantom and measuring them in a well-counter. The sensitivities measured according to the NEMA protocol for some recent PET scanners with both septa extended and retracted are shown in fig. 4.1.

The sensitivities have been corrected for scatter, with a scatter fraction measured according to the NEMA protocol (see below). The 3D sensitivities include all active lines-of-response (LORs), even though the number of LORs incorporated into the 3D reconstruction may be less in practice. The cylinder phantom used to measure sensitivity is generally longer (18.5 cm) than the axial FOV, and the 3D measurement may be affected by uncorrected scatter from the activity in those parts of the phantom outside the FOV.

As can be seen from fig. 4.1, retracting the septa results in a factor of about five increase in sensitivity after scatter correction. Two effects contribute to this increase: the removal of septa shadowing, and the increase in the number of active LORs. For example, for the ECAT 953B, the factor of 4.8 increase in sensitivity comprises factors of 1.9 for septa shadowing and 2.56 for the increase in the number of active LORs [Townsend et al., 1989]. Since 1990, the sensitivities of multi-ring scanners with septa extended have been in the range 3-6 cps/Bq/ml, increasing to 15-30 cps/Bq/ml with septa retracted. The ART and QUEST, tomographs without septa, have sensitivities of 7-10 cps/Bq/ml, exceeding that of full ring scanners such as the ECAT EXACT operated in 2D. The EXACT3D, the most sensitive commercial multi-ring scanner designed to date, has a sensitivity of 69 cps/Bq/ml.

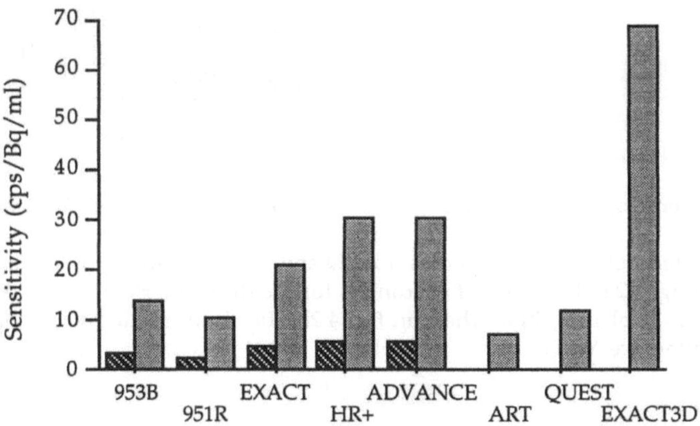

Figure 4.1 Comparative sensitivities for multi-ring and fully 3D scanners. Measurements have been obtained with a 20 cm diameter uniform cylinder containing an activity concentration less than 3.7 kBq/ml. Measurements for septa-retractable scanners are shown for 2D (black shading) and 3D (grey shading), and for the septaless scanners (ART, QUEST and EXACT3D) in 3D only.

The overall increase in sensitivity in 3D is, however, not distributed uniformly throughout the FOV. As a result of the truncated cylindrical geometry of the tomograph, the sensitivity is maximum in the centre of the axial FOV, decreasing towards either end. In fig. 4.2, the relative axial sensitivity profiles are shown for a 16-ring tomograph for (a) septa extended, and (b) septa retracted. In 2D, the direct and cross planes have slightly different sensitivities (fig. 4.2a). In 3D, the axial sensitivity profile peaks in the centre (fig. 4.2b), as expected from the cylindrical tomograph geometry. However, in practice, the largest ring difference (Δr) incorporated into the reconstruction is less than the maximum possible; for a 16-ring scanner, the maximum possible ring difference is ± 15, whereas the inclusion of ring differences of up to ± 11 results in a region of uniform axial sensitivity, as shown in this example between planes 8 and 24 (fig. 4.2b).

An alternative approach to the NEMA volume sensitivity estimate has been proposed by Bailey et al. [1991a] to provide an estimate of the *absolute* efficiency of the tomograph. The approach is based on measuring the count rate from an aluminium line source in air containing an accurately-known amount of radioactivity. The count rate is measured with different thickness (sleeves) of aluminium around the source, enabling the count rate for zero thickness to be estimated by extrapolation, thus correcting for the attenuation of radioactivity by the line source itself. This procedure, although not included in the original NEMA protocol, is a simple and straightforward approach to the measurement of absolute tomograph efficiency.

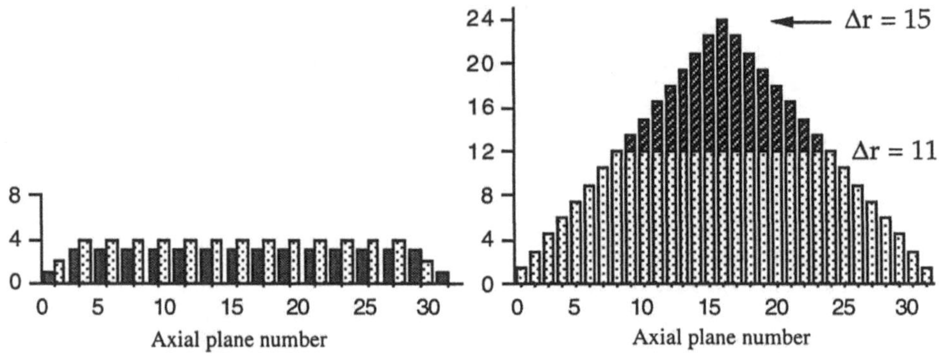

a) Septa extended, 2D acquisition (b) Septa retracted, 3D acquisition

Figure 4.2 Simulated relative sensitivities for 2D and 3D acquisitions as a function of axial plane number. In fig. 4.2a, the different shading is for the direct (dark shading; $\Delta r=2$) and cross (light shading; $\Delta r=3$) planes. Note that, in fig. 4.2b, the light shaded area corresponds to a maximum ring difference $\Delta r=11$.

SCATTER FRACTION

Compton scattering occurs when either one or both of the annihilation photons interact with an atomic electron in the tissue such that the photon loses energy and is deflected from its initial direction. Even though the scattered photons lose energy, the energy resolution of BGO is insufficient to reject all scatters, particularly those with small energy loss. In fact, even the energy resolution of NaI, which is better than that of BGO, is not sufficient to reject all scattered photons. When one or both photons scatter, the assumption that the two annihilation photons are collinear is then no longer valid and the event is assigned to an incorrect LOR. With septa extended, photons which scatter out of the plane are generally either eliminated by the septa or fall into LORs that are not acquired in 2D. In 3D, without septa, such scattered photons may be acquired, increasing the scatter fraction by a factor of about three, as shown in fig. 4.3 for a number of different scanners. Following the NEMA standard, the scatter fraction, defined as the ratio of scattered events to total events (T=trues+scatter), is measured with a line source of activity placed at three different radial positions (0 cm, 4 cm, and 8 cm) in a 20 cm diameter uniform water cylinder. The scatter fraction is generally higher at the centre of the phantom, and to account for the change in scatter fraction from the centre to the edge of the cylinder, an average scatter fraction (SF) is estimated by weighting the scatter counts S and total counts T at each source position by the area of the annulus at that radius:

$$SF = \frac{S(0) + 8 \cdot S(4) + 16 \cdot S(8)}{T(0) + 8 \cdot T(4) + 16 \cdot T(8)} \quad (4.1)$$

According to the NEMA protocol, both the (unscattered) trues and scatter are counted for a full axial FOV but for a centred, 24 cm diameter transaxial FOV. From levels of

10-15% in 2D, scatter fraction increases to 30-40% in 3D for all scanners; for accurate quantitation an appropriate scatter correction algorithm must be applied, as described in Chapter 3. Such algorithms are now successful in correcting scatter in 3D to levels below that encountered in 2D. The scatter fractions shown in fig. 4.3 are for a 20 cm diameter uniform cylinder. For the EXACT HR+, the SF for a 20 cm diameter cylinder is 37%, whereas for a 10 cm diameter cylinder SF is 21%. The scatter fraction for the brain will be in between these two values.

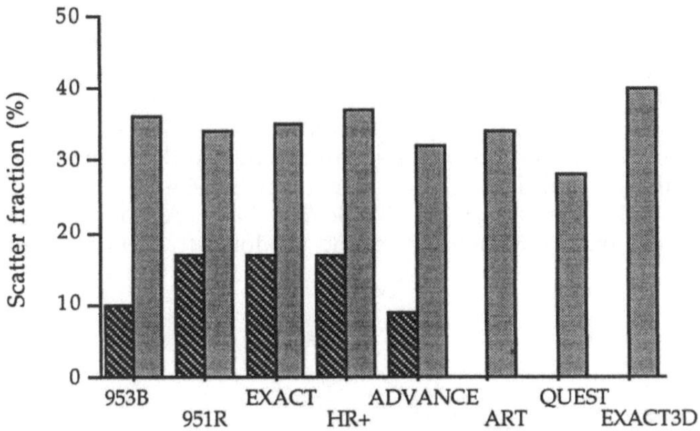

Figure 4.3 Comparison of scatter fraction for multi-ring and fully 3D scanners. Measurements have been obtained with a line source of activity and a 20 cm diameter uniform water cylinder according to the NEMA protocol. Measurements from septa-retractable scanners are shown for 2D (black shading) and 3D (grey shading), and for the septaless scanners (ART, QUEST and EXACT3D) in 3D only.

The magnitude of the scatter fraction is a function of the lower energy threshold that is applied to reject scattered events. Tomographs based on the BGO block detector have an energy resolution of about 25%, and are usually operated with an energy threshold in the range 250-350 keV. Many small-angle Compton scatters involve little energy loss and are therefore accepted within the wide energy window of BGO. New inorganic scintillators such as lutetium oxyorthosilicate (LSO) [Melcher and Schweitzer, 1992] have improved light output and better energy resolution that may help reduce the 3D scatter fraction. Nevertheless, the energy resolution of LSO will not be as good as that of NaI and, as seen with the QUEST scanner, even an energy resolution of 10-12% still results in a scatter fraction in 3D of around 30%.

COUNT RATE CAPABILITY

The count rate capability represents the response of the tomograph to changing activity levels in the FOV. In the absence of deadtime (DT) effects, the true coincidence count rate increases linearly with increasing activity. However, in practice, in a PET tomograph, as the activity in the FOV increases, deadtime in the detectors, electronics and acquisition system increases, limiting the observed true coincidence count rate. The most important contribution to DT arises from the intrinsic count rate capability of the detector, which is related to the slow decay time of the scintillators. A useful measure of the counting capability of the tomograph is the activity concentration at which deadtime reaches 50%. Percentage deadtime is defined as $(1-T/T_{ex})\cdot 100$, where T is the measured true coincidence rate (uncorrected for scatter) and T_{ex} is the expected trues rate based on a linear extrapolation from low count rates. For the EXACT HR+ the 50% DT level is reached in 2D with an activity concentration of 84 kBq/ml in 20 cm diameter cylinder (table 4.3), whereas in 3D, only 24 kBq/ml in the phantom is required to attain the 50% DT level.

It can be seen from fig. 4.4 that, for measurements with a 20 cm diameter cylinder, the maximum trues rate of 665 kcps in 3D is reached at a concentration of only 44 kBq/ml, whereas in 2D a maximum of 320 kcps is reached for a concentration over three times greater at 150 kBq/ml. This result illustrates an important advantage of 3D: high trues rates with low activity concentrations in the FOV. As expected, at concentrations above the peak, an increase in activity in the FOV actually results in a *reduction* in count rate as deadtime increases and the system becomes saturated. Randoms increase as the square of the activity in the FOV and, as can be seen from fig. 4.4, equal the trues rate at a concentration of 125 kBq/ml (2D) and 45 kBq/ml (3D). Although randoms rates are high in 3D, for a given true coincidence rate, the randoms fraction is smaller in 3D than 2D.

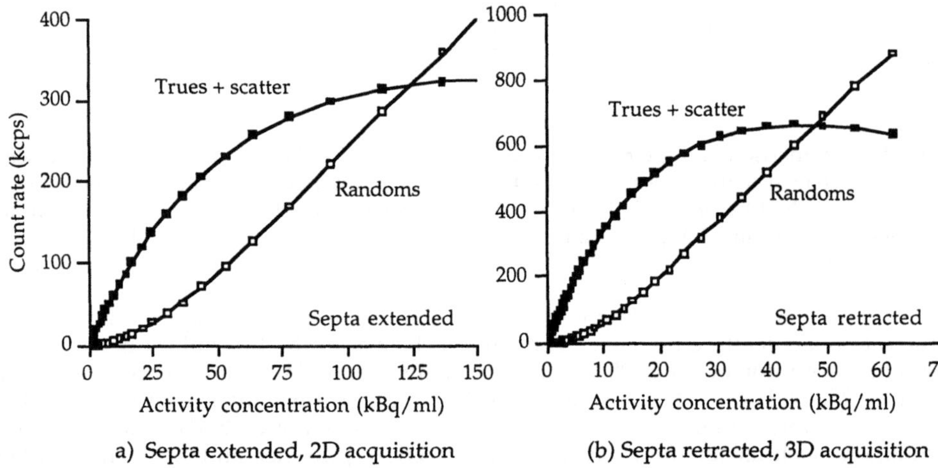

Figure 4.4 Trues+scatter and randoms rates for a multi-ring scanner with retractable septa (EXACT HR+). The count rates are measured with a 20 cm diameter uniform cylinder, with (a) septa extended and (b) septa retracted. The randoms rate is for a 24 cm FOV.

NOISE EQUIVALENT COUNT RATE

Overall, therefore, a higher true coincidence count rate can be achieved in 3D than in 2D, and the peak count rate is attained at a lower activity concentration in 3D than in 2D. However, with differing trues and randoms rates, and different levels of scatter in 2D and 3D, it is difficult to ascertain from curves such as those in fig. 4.4 the real advantages of 3D imaging. In order to more realistically assess these advantages, the concept of noise equivalent counts (NEC) has been proposed [Strother et al., 1990]. NEC is defined by the expression:

$$\mathrm{NEC} = \frac{[\mathrm{T} \cdot (1 - \mathrm{SF})]^2}{\mathrm{T} + 2\mathrm{fR}} \tag{4.2}$$

where T is the trues+scatter rate, R is the randoms rate, SF is the scatter fraction estimated according to equation 4.1, and f is the fraction of the maximum transaxial FOV subtended by a centred, 24 cm diameter field. The factor of two in the denominator comes from the subtraction of counts acquired in a delayed coincidence window to correct for randoms. NEC is a measure of global signal-to-noise, and has been used to evaluate the real improvement due to 3D [Bailey et al., 1991b].

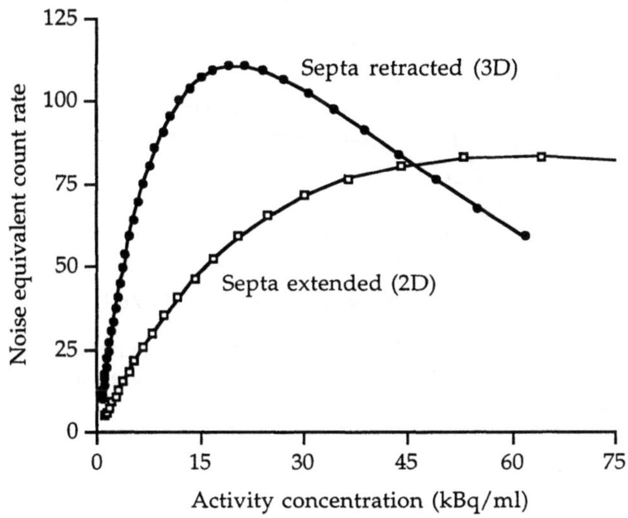

Figure 4.5 Noise equivalent count rate (NEC) for a multi-ring scanner with retractable septa (EXACT HR+). The measurements are for a 20 cm diameter uniform cylinder.

The NEC of a 20 cm diameter uniform cylinder measured in the EXACT HR+ with septa extended and retracted is shown in fig. 4.5. As expected from the behaviour of the true coincidence rate, the NEC in 3D reaches a maximum at a lower activity concentration (24 kBq/ml) than in 2D where the peak is not reached until the phantom contains an activity concentration of 75 kBq/ml, corresponding to over 350 MBq in the FOV. It is also interesting to note that the peak NEC is greater in 3D than in 2D for this tomograph.

It is evident from fig. 4.5 that the greatest increase in signal-to-noise is to be expected in the low activity concentration range, less than 24 kBq/ml. At higher concentrations the NEC in 3D starts to decline, until at around 45 kBq/ml, the 2D NEC actually exceeds the 3D NEC. At these and higher concentrations, the use of 3D is not indicated. It is important to realise that these results apply only to the phantom used for the measurements. Fig. 4.6 shows the 3D NEC for two different phantoms: uniform cylinders with 10 cm and 20 cm diameters. The NEC for the smaller phantom attains a greater maximum and at a higher activity concentration than the larger cylinder. Signal-to-noise estimates for more realistic, elliptical phantoms and human brain studies have been presented by Bailey [1996] with similar conclusions. Optimal performance in 3D is achieved with low activity concentrations in the FOV. This has led to changes in some PET protocols, notably in brain mapping studies where in 3D increased fractionation of the total radioactive dose into multiple small doses is to be preferred.

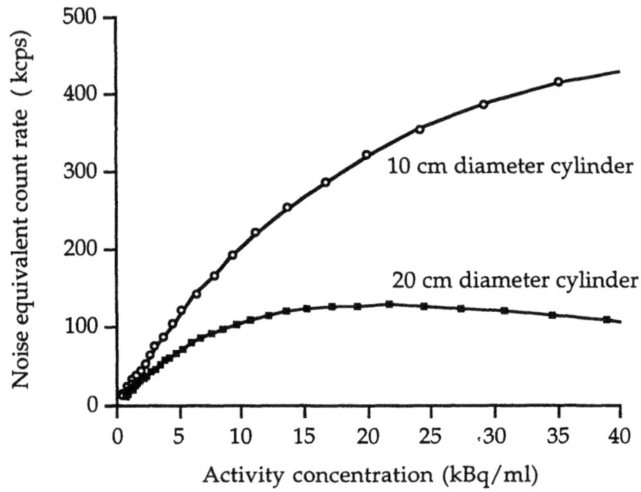

Figure 4.6 Noise equivalent count rate (NEC) for a multi-ring scanner (EXACT HR+) with septa retracted. The upper curve is for a 10 cm diameter uniform cylinder, and the lower curve for a 20cm diameter cylinder.

UNIFORMITY

Uniformity is a measure of the deviation of the tomograph from a uniform response by considering the reconstructed image of a uniform cylinder. The cylinder phantom containing a moderate amount of activity (to keep randoms and deadtime each below 20%) is placed in the scanner at a position 2.5 cm off-centre and imaged for a sufficient time to acquire an average of 20 million counts per slice. The data are corrected for detector normalization, deadtime, randoms, scatter and attenuation, as described in Chapter 3. According to the NEMA protocol, the reconstructed images are analysed by determining the number of counts in an array of contiguous 1 cm x 1 cm regions-of-interest (ROI) inscribed within a circle of diameter 18 cm centred on the image of the phantom in each slice. The negative and positive non-uniformities, NU- and NU+ respectively, are estimated for each slice according to the expressions [Karp et al., 1991]:

$$NU+ = \frac{+(C_{max} - C_{avg})}{C_{avg}}$$

$$NU- = \frac{-(C_{avg} - C_{min})}{C_{avg}} \qquad (4.3)$$

where C_{max} and C_{min} are the maximum and minimum number of counts within any square ROI in the slice, and C_{ave} is the average number of counts over all the regions within the slice. The volume non-uniformity can be estimated in a similar way by performing these calculations for each slice and then averaging over all slices. As can be seen from table 4.3, the volume variance shows no significant differences between 2D and 3D, although for the EXACT HR+, the 2D uniformity appears slightly better than in 3D.

OUT-OF-FIELD ACTIVITY

One of the most difficult problems to address in 3D PET is the increase in scatter and randoms arising from activity outside the FOV. In 2D, single photons originating from this activity and entering the FOV are prevented from reaching the detectors by the septa. In 3D, the tomograph is unshielded and such photons will contribute to increased detector deadtime and increased randoms. Coincidence events from activity just outside the FOV may be detected if one or both of the annihilation photons scatter into the detectors. The importance of this effect will depend upon the relative amounts of activity inside and outside the FOV, the design of the shielding on the front and rear of the tomograph, and the geometry of the tomograph (fig. 3.18).

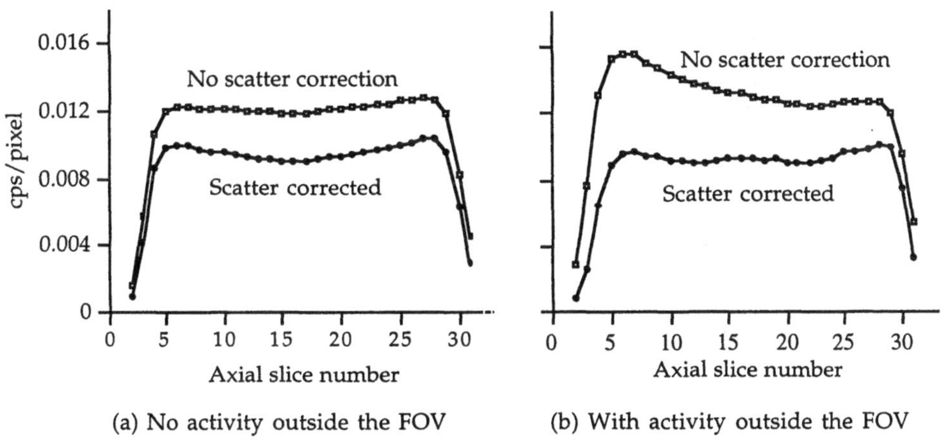

Figure 4.7 Mean ROI values for reconstructed images of a uniform cylinder, imaged with (a) only activity in the cylinder, and (b) with activity in the cylinder and in a smaller cylinder located immediately outside the FOV. The vertical scale is the same for both graphs.

The effect of increased scatter is illustrated in fig. 4.7 with reconstructed images of a uniform cylinder of activity imaged both with and without additional activity located immediately outside the FOV. In both cases, the cylinder was imaged, reconstructed and a circular ROI drawn on the image of the cylinder in each slice. The mean activity value in each ROI is shown in fig. 4.7 as a function of axial slice number. In the absence of activity outside the FOV, the expected behaviour is observed (fig. 4.7a): a similar contribution in each slice due to scatter from activity in the FOV which is corrected by one of the standard methods (Chapter 3). In this example, the dual-energy window approach [Grootoonk et al., 1992] was used. Fig. 4.7b shows the same analysis performed on phantom data acquired with a small cylinder of activity positioned immediately outside the FOV. The total activity in the small cylinder was five times greater than the activity in the phantom in the FOV. Due to the end shielding of the scanner, there is an increase in the ROI mean value with *increasing* distance from the external source, which in this example was placed close to plane 31 (fig. 4.7b). This increasing mean value is due to the contribution of scatter from the activity outside the FOV. The dual-energy window scatter correction algorithm successfully corrects for this additional contribution, which represented a 60% increase in scatter in planes 4-8. Other scatter correction algorithms may not account for out-of-field activity.

An effect of out-of-field activity which is potentially more significant than the increased scatter component, is the reduction in NEC due to the increased randoms rates. Bailey [1996] observed that with a uniform cylinder phantom, the NEC was reduced by 50% by placing an additional 5 litre cylinder of activity immediately outside the field of view, even though the effect of the increased deadtime and randoms on the expected count rate from the phantom in the FOV was only 17%.

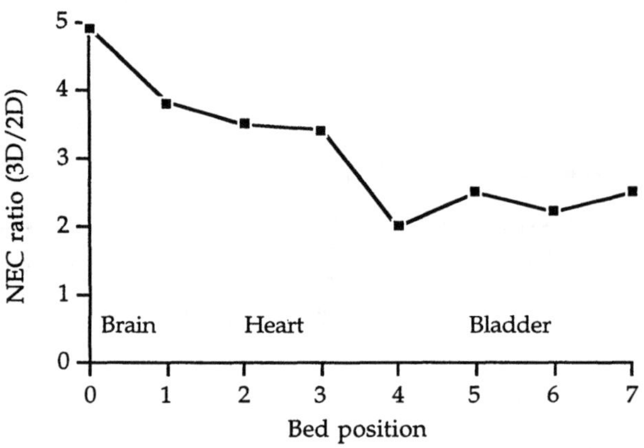

Figure 4.8 The ratio of 3D NEC to 2D NEC for data acquired during a whole body FDG PET scan. At each of the eight bed positions, the NEC was calculated according to equation 4.2 with appropriate values for SF and f. The ratio represents the improvement in signal-to-noise of 3D relative to 2D.

Out-of-field activity is potentially a serious problem for whole body imaging in 3D (see Chapter 5: Whole Body Imaging in 3D). For the brain, additional lead shielding can be introduced into the patient port of the tomograph, effectively reducing the single photon flux from out-of-field activity [Grootoonk et al., 1996]. For whole body imaging, additional shielding is not possible due to the changing body size and shape as the patient is stepped through the scanner. Fig. 4.8 illustrates the significant reduction in NEC that arises in 3D from out-of-field activity in the brain, heart and bladder during an FDG whole body PET scan. The scan was performed on the same subject in 2D and 3D and a global NEC estimated at each bed position using appropriate values for the scatter fraction and f in equation 4.2. The ratio of the 3D NEC to 2D NEC is then plotted for each bed position, as shown in fig. 4.8. The highest ratio, a factor five, occurs with the brain in the FOV, as expected from the results presented earlier for cylinder phantoms. This factor decreases to four in the region of the heart, and then decreases to a factor of only two in the abdomen because of the increasing randoms rate due to out-of-field activity in the brain, heart and bladder. Signal-to-noise is proportional to the square root of the NEC [Strother et al., 1990], and therefore 3D imaging in the abdomen represents at best only a 40% improvement in signal-to-noise. This observation has some implications for the performance of the fully 3D tomographs such as the ART and the QUEST that target clinical applications, and whole body imaging in particular.

SUMMARY

The physical performance parameters of septa-retractable PET tomographs and fully 3D tomographs are summarized in tables 4.3 and 4.4, respectively. It is important to realize that summarizing tomograph performance for the purposes of comparison is complex, and the conclusions drawn from such an exercise must be interpreted with caution. All performance figures contain a level of uncertainty related to the number of different parameters upon which they are based. These parameters include factors such as the energy discrimination level (LLD), the extent of the transaxial and axial FOV, the maximum ring difference used for 3D acquisition, and the coincidence time window and electronics-related settings. A knowledge of the exact dimensions of the phantoms used for the measurements is important because a 5 mm variation in wall thickness leads to a 10% variation in photon attenuation. Uncertainties in the radioactivity assay (with well-counter or dose calibrator) will directly affect the performance assessment.

		ECAT 953B		EXACT HR+		ADVANCE	
		2D	3D	2D	3D	2D*	3D
In-plane resolution (mm)	r=1 cm	5.8	6.0	4.5 x 4.5	4.5 x 4.7	4.5 x 5.0	4.5 x 5.0
(tangential x radial)	r=10cm	6.0 x 6.4		4.5 x 6.0	4.5 x 6.0	5.0 x 5.5	5.0 x 6.0
Axial resolution (mm)	r=0 cm	4.2	5.2	3.9	3.9	4.0	6.0
	r=10cm	5.8	6.3	4.8	5.3	5.5	6.5
Trues sensitivity (cps/Bq/ml)		2.9	13.8	5.7	30.4	5.7	30.4
Scatter fraction (%)		10	36	17	37	10	34
Activity at 50% DT (kBq/ml)		90		84	24	181	31
Peak NEC (kcps)		74	52	84	110	261	159
Activity at peak (kBq/ml)		100	22.2	130	24.1	152	24
Volume uniformity (%)		5	5	3.9	5		4

Table 4.3 Performance parameters of PET scanners with retractable septa. * These values are for the high sensitivity mode of the ADVANCE in 2D. Note the transaxial resolution is an average over the central axial planes.

This summary is an attempt to highlight, in particular, the differing performance in 2D and 3D of the septa-retractable tomographs, and allows a comparison of the 3D capabilities of all tomographs, both septa retractable and fully 3D. Overall, 3D offers significant gains in sensitivity which, in most imaging situations, are reflected in improved count rates and signal-to-noise in the images. No significant loss of either in-plane or axial spatial resolution is observed, except for the ADVANCE in 3D where the non-uniform detector sampling results in a degradation of axial resolution. In 2D, however, the 8 mm crystal size combined with a low scatter fraction leads to a large peak NEC at higher activity levels than in 3D. The increased count rates in 3D place increased demands on the deadtime performance of the tomographs, suggesting that lower injected activities are to be preferred in 3D. The greatest increase in noise equivalent counts, and hence image signal-to-noise, is observed at low activity concentrations. The maximum NEC in 3D occurs at activity concentrations 3-6 times smaller than in 2D. An increased axial FOV results in an improved maximum NEC in 3D [Karp et al.,1993] compared with 2D. Finally, although the scatter fraction increases by a factor of three over 2D, effective scatter correction algorithms now exist (see Chapter 3) to ensure accurate quantitation in 3D.

		ECAT ART	QUEST	EXACT 3D
In-plane resolution (mm)	r=1 cm	5.7 x 6.0	5.5	4.7
(radial x tangential)	r=10 cm	6.4 x 6.7	5.8	4.7 x 6.5
Axial resolution (mm)	r=0 cm	6.0	6	5.2
	r=10 cm	7.2	6	6.3
Trues sensitivity (cps/Bq/ml)		7.5	12.2	69.0
Scatter fraction (%)		37	28	40
Peak NEC (kcps)		27	30	173
Activity at peak (kBq/ml)		14.7	7.0	6.9

Table 4.4 Performance parameters of fully 3D PET scanners

In this section, tomograph performance in 3D has been compared with the standard performance characteristics in 2D. However, the acquisition of increased amounts of data in 3D presents additional challenges for data storage and image reconstruction. These issues will be examined in the following sections.

Three Dimensional Data Sets

The advent of 3D PET was accompanied by a significant increase in the size of the acquired data sets, typically an increase of at least an order of magnitude. This section describes some of the problems associated with these large data sets, the solutions that have been proposed and implemented and the current status.

DATA SET SIZES

In a period of some seventeen years, from 1979 to 1996, the size of the data sets acquired by multi-ring PET tomographs increased from 363 LORs in the ECAT II to approximately 200 million in the EXACT3D. This progression, spanning over six orders of magnitude, is summarized in fig. 4.9. Over the eleven years from 1979 to 1990, the number of acquired LORs increased by a factor of a thousand, whereas in the five years from 1990 to 1994 the data set sizes increased by a further factor of a thousand. It is interesting to speculate whether the logarithmic increase in data set size with time shown in fig. 4.9 will continue in the future. The major impact of 3D is first seen in 1990 with the ECAT 953B, where a factor of eight increase in the number of LORs acquired in 3D compared to 2D occurred. Multi-ring scanners with retractable septa followed the 953B with factors of 10-20 times more data acquired in 3D than in 2D.

Evidently, the storage and transfer of such large data sets presented a problem to the standard data acquisition configuration designed to handle 2D data sets. Data acquisition memory and disk capacity was rapidly exceeded by the large 3D data sets, and provision had to be made to increase resources. Fortunately, increased memory and storage capacity has not been a significant financial issue owing to the rapidly declining costs and increasing size of computer memory and magnetic disks, and the availability of magneto-optical disk storage and high capacity, compact tape systems. Currently, acquisition memory up to 512 Mbytes is available on state-of-the-art tomographs, with direct on-line sinogram storage capacity exceeding 20 Gbytes. High capacity off-line storage is also available with the emergence of 23 Gbyte disks at low cost.

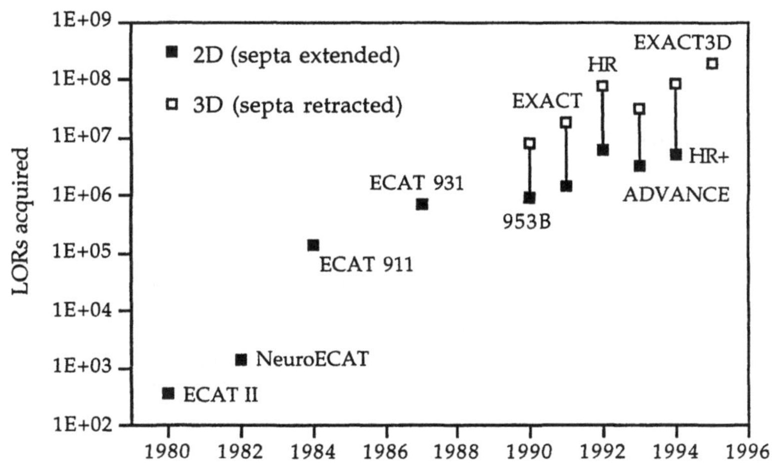

Figure 4.9 The increasing size of acquired data sets over the period 1979-1996. Both 2D (filled squares) and 3D (empty squares) data sets are shown. Septa retractable scanners are shown with a vertical line joining the 2D and 3D data set sizes. Earlier scanners (1987 and before) are 2D only, and the EXACT3D (1996) is 3D only. Note the logarithmic scale for the ordinate; data sizes have increased by six orders of magnitude over the seventeen-year period shown.

Current sinogram sizes in 2D and 3D are listed in table 4.5 for some recent PET tomographs. With the exception of the EXACT HR that has high in-plane sampling, typical 2D sinogram data set sizes are in the range 3-6 Mbytes per time frame. As expected, in 3D, these sizes increase by at least a factor of ten, up to 30-170 Mbytes per frame. Without compression, a 20-frame dynamic ligand study on the HR+ would require 3.4 Gbytes of data storage. Even with the state-of-the-art technology supplied with the tomograph, the necessary cost limitations on medical imaging equipment result in the management of such large data sets being impractical in a clinical environment.

To make 3D PET a practical methodology, advantage must be taken of over-sampling in the tomograph to introduce some on-line compression techniques. When techniques such as projection averaging (Chapter 2: axial and transaxial mashing) are used, sinogram data sets can be reduced to 10-20 Mbytes per frame with minimal loss of resolution, particularly for brain imaging. By providing on-line data compression, acquisition memory, back-up tape storage and off-line disk capacity requirements can all be relaxed.

	2D	3D (full)	3D (compressed)
ECAT 951R	2.9	24.6	8.2
EXACT EXACT	2.8	34.5	13.9
EXACT HR	12.1	148.4	28.5
EXACT HR+	5.2	170.0	19.8
ADVANCE	6.5	60.0	24.0

Table 4.5 Sizes of data sets (Mbytes) in 2D, full 3D and compressed 3D

LIST MODE ACQUISITION

Since 3D sinogram data sets are approaching or exceeding 100 Mbytes per frame, the acquisition of very short (5-10 sec) time frames, during which up to a maximum of 3-6 million events are collected, makes very inefficient use of the on-line memory and data storage. At best, only one in five sinogram elements will contain an event. A similar observation for time-of-flight (TOF) PET also led to the implementation of list mode acquisition, ensuring an efficient use of memory on scanners with access to TOF information. In addition, in situations where decisions on spatial and temporal sampling cannot be made prior to the study, list mode acquisition offers an alternative approach. In list mode acquisition, the information related to the detector pair corresponding to a coincident event is explicitly stored. The acquired data is stored not as formatted sinograms but as a list of individual event words, interleaved with 100 msec time stamps. Upon completion of the acquisition, the list mode data can be 'replayed' into sinograms with the required spatial and temporal sampling for reconstruction.

The size of the list mode data file will depend upon the data rate and the overall imaging time. List mode offers the capability of exploring finer temporal sampling, and for short frame times acquired at moderate acquisition rates, makes more efficient use of the storage capacity. For example, for the EXACT HR+, a 5 sec time frame acquired without on-line compression at a rate of 400 kcps will occupy 170 Mbytes of disk space. The same data, collected in list mode, and assuming a 20% randoms rate, will occupy only 5.6 Mbytes.

Prior to the availability of on-line sinogram formatting, PET data were acquired in list mode and formatted into sinograms off-line. The availability of specific hardware for on-line sinogram formation led to the disappearance of the list mode capability. However, the recent emergence of fully 3D tomographs such as the EXACT3D with a 382 Mb (uncompressed) single frame size has led to a revival of the list mode capability.

List mode hardware is currently available for the EXACT3D, HR+ and HR range of PET tomographs.

Three-Dimensional Reconstruction

In addition to the difficulties presented by the large 3D data sets, fully three-dimensional reconstruction is a computationally intensive procedure owing to the large number of LORs that are backprojected through the imaging volume (Chapter 2). The hardware and software to perform this task have improved considerably since the appearance of the first septa-retractable scanner in 1990. This section examines some of the progress of the last eight years, and summarizes the current status.

HARDWARE FOR 3D RECONSTRUCTION

Originally, the difficulty of developing 3D methodology was substantially increased by the long reconstruction times required for the 3D reprojection algorithm (Chapter 2) to complete on a SparcStation 1. Progressively, since 1990, improvements in hardware performance and parallel implementation of the algorithms, has led to a considerable reduction in the reconstruction timings, as shown in fig. 4.10. From the approximately eight hours required to reconstruct a 128 x 128 x 31 image volume on a Sparc 1 from a total of 7 million LORs, reconstruction times of 8-10 min can now be achieved for images of 128 x 128 x 63 from 20 million LORs. The reasons for this progress include improvements in hardware performance, an efficient (microcoded) parallel implementation of the reprojection algorithm on an array of processors, and on-line compression to limit the number of LORs to be backprojected.

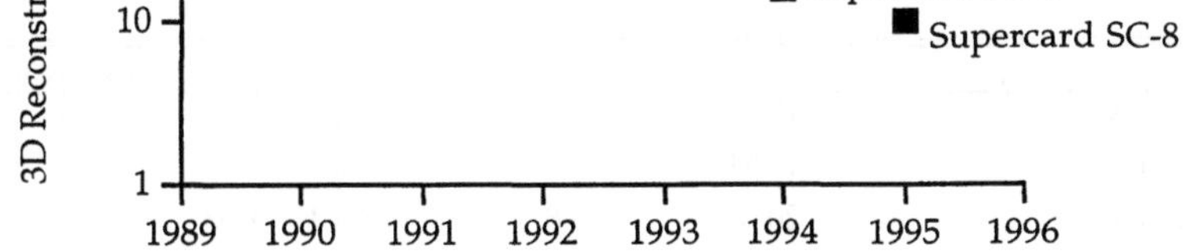

Figure 4.10 Reconstruction timings for the 3D reprojection algorithm showing the significant improvement since the first implementation on a SparcStation 1.

To achieve reconstruction times of ten minutes or less, both the EXACT and ADVANCE range of scanners offer arrays of i860 processors operating in parallel, as shown schematically in fig. 4.11. The EXACT HR+, for example, is provided with two quad Supercard boards (CSP Inc., Billerica, MA), each board equipped with four i860 processors. A parallel implementation of the reprojection algorithm assigns groups of

2D projections (see Chapter 2) to separate processors for filtering and subsequent backprojection into a shared image volume. Increasing the number of processors results in the reconstruction time eventually becoming dominated by the inter-processor communication speed rather than the computing cycle time of the individual processors. Increasing the number of processors beyond the eight currently provided on the HR+ is of little benefit in reducing the reconstruction time for each frame. At a level of ten minutes per frame, including all quantitative corrections, 3D PET can be considered a practical methodology.

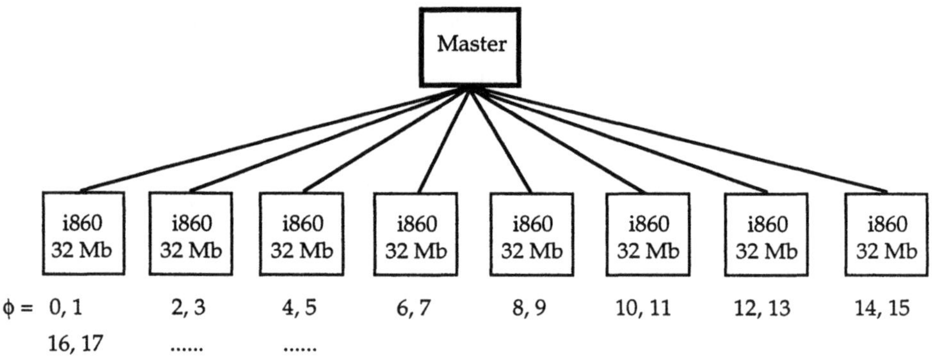

Figure 4.11 Schematic of the hardware for a parallel implementation of the 3D reprojection algorithm on an array of eight i860 processors. Projections in different directions (such as ϕ =0,1 and 2,3 ...) are assigned to different i860s and processed in parallel.

Reconstruction times for the different scanners, the number of available processors and the number of LORs to be backprojected are summarised in table 4.6. Supercard hardware is provided standard in the acquisition and computing system of the EXACT, ART and ADVANCE tomographs. However, impressive reconstruction times are now being achieved on a range of fast, low-cost, Pentium-based desktop processors. It is anticipated that such low-cost, general-purpose computers will replace the dedicated, i860-based processors that are currently used for 3D.

	No. LORs	No. of i860s	Image size	Time (min)
ECAT EXACT	13 M	4	128 x 128 x 47	10
EXACT HR	19 M	8	128 x 128 x 47	10
EXACT HR+	20 M	8	128 x 128 x 63	9
ADVANCE	24 M	9	128 x 128 x 35	8

Table 4.6 Reconstruction timings for the 3D reprojection algorithm implemented on different scanners

SOFTWARE FOR 3D RECONSTRUCTION

The 3D reprojection algorithm [Kinahan and Rogers, 1989] is the standard algorithm for 3D reconstruction that has been implemented on the i860-based parallel processors, shown schematically in fig. 4.11. Implementations for SparcStations and Pentium processors have also been developed. Mathematical details of the reprojection algorithm are given in Chapter 2. Algorithms that rebin a 3D data set into a 2D set offer an alternative approach which reduces reconstruction time by allowing a 2D reconstruction algorithm to be used on the rebinned 3D data set. Rebinning algorithms, also described in Chapter 2, include single-slice rebinning [Daube-Witherspoon and Muehllehner, 1987], and multi-slice rebinning [Lewitt et al., 1994]. Single-slice rebinning has been used in particular to provide fast 2D reconstruction of 3D data sets to verify patient positioning and check the integrity of the acquired data. However, single-slice rebinning leads to artifacts in the reconstructed image, and multi-slice rebinning results in noise amplification. Recently, Fourier rebinning [Defrise et al., 1997] has been proposed as an alternative approach that avoids the artifacts and noise amplification of the other rebinning methods. Software to perform Fourier rebinning is now integrated into the image reconstruction package for tomographs such as the EXACT HR+.

A major advantage of a rebinning method that noiselessly rebins a 3D data set into a 2D data set is that 2D statistical methods can then be applied to reconstruct the images. One such iterative method, Ordered-Subset EM (OSEM) [Hudson and Larkin, 1994], has been used successfully in combination with Fourier rebinning [Kinahan et al., 1996]. Software is now generally available for OSEM, and to a limited extent, for other statistical approaches such as the penalized weighted least squares (PWLS) algorithm proposed by Fessler [1994], and efforts to apply these techniques to 3D PET data are in progress [Comtat et al., 1998]. In view of the significant improvement in image quality that can be achieved by statistical reconstruction methods, an approach such as Fourier rebinning and OSEM now offers a practical alternative to the widely-used 3D reprojection algorithm.

Conclusion

While earlier chapters developed appropriate methodology for 3D PET, image reconstruction and quantitation, this chapter presents a review of the instrumentation performance for acquisition, reconstruction and management of 3D data sets. Particular importance is placed on comparing 3D performance with standard 2D methodology in order to highlight the advantages and challenges of 3D and to emphasize the applications for which 3D is especially suited. The range and complexity of the different procedures for accurate quantitation in 3D reflects the extensive research and development resources that have been devoted to these issues in recent years. This research has contributed significantly to both improving and understanding the technology, and to introducing 3D as a practical methodology. These developments are on-going, leading to continual improvement in tomograph performance, image quality, quantitative accuracy, reconstruction timing, and management of the data acquisition and storage.

The wider availability of list mode data acquisition may lead to improved scatter correction by providing access to the individual photon energy. Spatial resolution improvements can be anticipated from smaller detectors, and the increased sensitivity of 3D will lead to higher image statistics and hence less smoothing will be required during the reconstruction. Tracking systems will monitor subject movement throughout the scan and accurately correct for intra-scan motion. The introduction of new inorganic scintillators such as LSO, with fast scintillation decay and improved light output

[Melcher and Schweitzer, 1992] and the development of faster electronics, will improve the noise equivalent count performance of current BGO-based tomographs, particularly in 3D.

Three-dimensional acquisition for PET offers significant advantages over the standard, well-understood, 2D methodology for an increasing number of research and clinical applications. However, there is an urgent need to redesign the familiar, standard protocols in order to fully assess the advantages of 3D and to exploit the benefits. Specific 3D protocols have been developed at a number of PET centres with access to septa-retractable, or fully 3D, tomographs. The next chapter will review several of these protocols, and describe the associated research and clinical applications for which 3D PET methodology has been identified as offering significant advantages.

References

Bailey DL, Jones T, Spinks TJ. A method for measuring the absolute sensitivity of positron emission tomographic scanners. Eur J Nucl Med 1991a;18:374-379.

Bailey DL, Jones T, Spinks TJ, Gilardi MC, Townsend DW. Noise equivalent count measurements in a Neuro-PET scanner with retractable septa. IEEE Trans Med Imag 1991b;10(3):256-260.

Bailey DL, Young H, Bloomfield PM, Meikle SR, Glass D, Myers MJ, Spinks TJ, Watson CC, Luk P, Peters M, Jones T. ECAT ART - a continuosly rotating PET camera: performance characteristics, inital clinical studies, and installation considerations in a nuclear medicine department. Eur J Nucl Med 1997;24(1):5-15.

Bailey DL, Meikle SR, Jones T. Effective sensitivity in 3D PET: The impact of detector dead time on 3D system performance. IEEE Trans Nucl Sci 1997;44 (3):1180-1185.

Bailey DL. Quantification in 3D positron emission tomography. [PhD Thesis]. Department of Physics, University of Surrey, 1996.

Brix G, Zaers J, Adam L-E, Bellemann ME, Ostertag H, Trojan H, Haberkorm U, Doll J, Oberdorfer F, Lorenz WJ. Performance evaluation of a whole-body PET scanner using the NEMA protocol. J Nucl Med 1997;38(10):1614-1623.

Colsher JG. Fully three-dimensional positron emission tomography. Phys Med Biol 1980;20:103-115.

Comtat C, Kinahan PE, Defrise M, Michel C, Townsend DW. Fast reconstruction of 3D PET data with accurate statistical modeling. IEEE Medical Imaging Conference Record 1998. To appear.

Daube-Witherspoon ME and Muehllehner G. Treatment of axial data in three-dimensional PET. J Nucl Med 1987;28:1717-1724.

DeGrado TR, Turkington TG, Williams JJ, Stearns CW, Hoffman JM, Coleman RE. Performance characteristics of a whole-body PET scanner. J Nucl Med 1994;35:1398-1406.

Defrise M, Kinahan PE, Townsend DW, Michel C, Sibomana M, Newport D. Exact and approximate rebinning algorithms for 3D PET data. IEEE Trans Med Imag 1997;16(2):145-158.

Derenzo SE, Moses WW, Huesman RH, Budinger TF. Critical instrumentation issues for resolution smaller than 2 mm, high sensitivity brain PET. In: Uemura K, Lassen NA, Jones T, Kanno I, editors. Quantification of Brain Function. Tracer Kinetics and Image Analysis in Brain PET. Excerpta Medica, 1993: 25-37.

Fessler JA. Penalized weighted least-squares image reconstruction for Positron Emission Tomography. IEEE Trans Med Imag 1994;13(2):1994.

Grootoonk S, Spinks TJ, Jones T, Michel C, Bol A. Correction for scatter using a dual energy window technique with a tomograph operating without septa. IEEE Medical Imaging Conference Record 1992;2:1569-1573.

Grootoonk S, Fink G, Brun T. Impact of a neuro-insert on brain scanning with the ECAT EXACT HR+ PET Scanner. Neuroimage 1996;3(3):S25.

Hudson HM and Larkin RS. Accelerated image reconstruction using ordered subsets of projection data. IEEE Trans Med Imag 1994;13(4):601-609.

Jones T, Bailey DL, Bloomfield PM, Spinks TJ, Jones W, Vaigneur K, Reed J, Young J, Newport D, Moyers C, Casey ME, Nutt R.. Performance characteristics and novel design aspects of the most sensitive PET camera built for high temporal and spatial resolution. J Nucl Med 1996;37(5):85P.

Karp JS, Daube-Witherspoon ME, Hoffman EJ, Lewellen TK, Links JM, Wong WH, Hichwa RD, Casey ME, Colsher JG, Hitchens RE, Muehllehner G, Stoub EW. Performance standards in Positron Emission Tomography. J Nucl Med 1991;32(12):2342-2350.

Karp JS, Kinahan PE, Muehllehner G, Countryman P. Effect of increased axial field of view on the performance of a volume PET scanner. IEEE Trans Med Imag 1993;12(2):299-306.

Kinahan PE and Rogers JG. Analytic three-dimensional image reconstruction using all detected events. IEEE Trans Nucl Sci 1989;NS-36:964-968.

Kinahan PE, Michel C, Defrise M, Townsend DW, Sibomana M, Lonnux M, Newport DF, Luketich JD. Fast iterative reconstruction of 3D PET data. IEEE Medical Imaging Conference Record 1996;3:1918-1922.

Lewellen TK, Kohlmyer SG, Miyaoka RS, Schubert S, Stearns CW. Investigation of count rate performance of the General Electric ADVANCE positron emission tomograph. IEEE Trans Nucl Sci 1995;42:1051-1057.

Lewellen TK, Kohlmyer SG, Miyaoka RS, Kaplan MS. Investigation of the performance of the General Electric ADVANCE positron emission tomograph in 3D mode. IEEE Trans Nucl Sci 1996;43:2199-2206.

Lewitt RM, Muehllehner G, Karp JS. Three-dimensional image recontruction for PET by multi-slice rebinning and axial image filtering. Phys Med Biol 1994;39(3):321-339.

Mazoyer B, Trebossen R, Deutch R, Casey M, Blohm K. Physical characteristics of the ECAT 953B/31: A new high resolution brain positron tomograph. IEEE Trans Med Imag 1991;10(4):499-504.

Melcher CL and Schweitzer JS. Cerium-doped lutetium oxyorthosilicate: a fast, efficient new scintillator. IEEE Trans Nucl Sci 1992;39(4):502-505.

Muehllehner G. Positron camera with extended counting rate capability. J Nucl Med 1975;16:653-657.

Spinks TJ, Jones T, Bailey DL, Townsend DW, Grootoonk S, Bloomfield PM, Gilardi MC, Casey ME, Sipe B, Reed J. Physical performance of a positron tomograph for brain imaging with retractable septa. Phys Med Biol 1992;37:1637-1655.

Spinks TJ, Bailey DL, Bloomfield PM, Miller M, Murayama H, Jones T, Jones W, Reed J, Newport D, Casey ME, Nutt R. Performance of a new 3D-only PET scanner - the EXACT3D. IEEE Medical Imaging Conference Record 1997;2:1275-1284.

Strother SC, Casey ME, Hoffman EJ. Measuring PET scanner sensitivity: relating countrates to image signal-to-noise ratios using noise equivalent counts. IEEE Trans Nucl Sci 1990;37(2):783-788.

Townsend DW, Frey P, Jeavons AP, Reich G, Tochon-Danguy HJ, Donath A, Christin A, Schaller G. High density avalanche chamber (HIDAC) positron camera. J Nucl Med 1987;28:1554-1562.

Townsend DW, Spinks TJ, Jones T, Geissbuhler A, Defrise M, Gilardi MC, Heather J. Three-dimensional reconstruction of PET data from a multi-ring camera. IEEE Trans Nucl Sci 1989;36:1056-1065.

Wienhard K, Eriksson L, Grootoonk S, Casey M, Pietrzyk U, Heiss W-D. Performance evaluation of the positron scanner ECAT EXACT. J Comput Assist Tomogr 1992;16(5):804-813.

Wienhard K, Dahlbom M, Eriksson L, Michel C, Bruckbauer T, Pietrzyk U, Heiss WD. The ECAT EXACT HR: performance of a new high resolution positron scanner. J Comput Assist Tomogr 1994;18:110-118.

Chapter 5. APPLICATIONS OF 3D PET

Klaus Wienhard
Max-Planck-Institut für neurologische Forschung, Köln, Germany

With contributions from:

DL Bailey, A Bol, DJ Brooks, T Bruckbauer, PD Cutler L Eriksson, L Farde, S Grootoonk, WD Heiss, T Jones, K Herholz, M Ingvar, C Michel, MP Miller, PK Morrish, U Pietrzyk, JS Rakshi, P Remy, A Thiel, R. Trébossen, and AG De Volder

Introduction

This chapter presents examples of the application of 3D PET in research and clinical studies. The contributions have been selected as representative of the types of applications for which 3D methodology is important. However, no attempt has been made to cover the entire range of applications for which 3D methodology could be used. This chapter is rather an overview of how different laboratories apply 3D PET. In a number of PET Centres, the use of 3D has become routine, particularly for brain studies. Thus, those difficulties which were considered major obstacles for 3D a few years ago have now been, to a large extent, resolved. These difficulties include the increased scatter contribution, high count rates, large data files, long reconstruction times, and absolute quantitation. The contributions in this chapter discuss many of these issues, and demonstrate how scan protocols have been optimized to take advantage of the benefits of 3D, how they compare with standard 2D PET, and to what extent the same results are obtained in 3D as in 2D.

In particular, examples are presented of studies in which the higher efficiency in 3D leads to better signal-to-noise in images that can be reconstructed with less smoothing. An area in which the increased efficiency in 3D has had a major impact is in brain mapping studies. Activation protocols optimized for 3D have led to increased statistical power (more task repeats), and allowed, for the first time, cerebral activation to be mapped with PET in single individuals. One of the most widespread applications of PET is to the measurement of cerebral glucose metabolism by the FDG method. Optimized FDG protocols have been developed for 3D, and the results compared with 2D. Accurate estimates of glucose metabolism have been obtained from studies performed in 3D with factors of up to three reduction in injected dose. Improved image quality at lower injected dose is a major advantage of 3D with considerable potential for pediatric applications. In particular, the ability to quantitatively measure cerebral

B. Bendriem and D.W. Townsend (eds.) The Theory and Practice of 3D PET, 133-167.

blood flow and glucose metabolism in the developing brain by the administration of very low radioactive doses could have a major impact in pediatric neurology. Increased resolution and signal-to-noise are also important in presurgical tumour studies in adults, allowing improved delineation of tumour extent.

Although challenging the data acquisition and storage capacity of most tomographs, kinetic studies performed in 3D have led to increased accuracy in modelling, and lower variance on rate constants with no evidence of bias. Quantitative analysis in neurodegenerative disorders such as Parkinson's disease has shown improved modelling accuracy with 3D data sets.

Most of the applications described in this chapter are for the brain. The development of 3D methodology has been largely oriented towards cerebral studies where issues such as correction for increased scatter have been successfully addressed. For the remainder of the body, the situation is not quite so favourable. Increased levels of scatter are encountered, and the algorithms described in Chapter 3 are less successful than they are for the brain. The performance of the scanner is degraded by scatter and randoms from activity outside the FOV (Chapter 4). Cardiac imaging in 3D is in its infancy, particularly when quantitation is required as in the case of myocardial blood flow measurements. This topic will not be covered here. However, whole body imaging in 3D is an important application area because of the clinical significance of whole body imaging and the fact that both the ECAT ART and the QUEST, which specifically target clinical whole body imaging, are 3D only tomographs. A description of appropriate 3D whole body imaging protocols is included in this chapter, showing how the protocols may be optimized to eliminate artifacts and achieve uniform axial resolution and signal-to-noise.

The contributions presented in this chapter demonstrate the widespread applicability of 3D methodology to PET, and amply justify the engineering and technological effort that has been devoted in the past few years to addressing and solving the problems. The group of applications presented here was selected by investigators at the various PET centers to give an impression of both the current impact of 3D in PET, and the enormous potential that still remains to be exploited.

Experience of 3D PET at the Karolinska Hospital, Stockholm, Sweden

INTRODUCTION

The Karolinska group has two positron camera systems, an ECAT EXACT HR and an ECAT EXACT 31. Both tomographs can presently be operated in 3D and are almost entirely run with 3D protocols. Only 15% are still conventional 2D studies. The ECAT EXACT HR system has high spatial resolution, 3.6 mm FWHM transaxially and 4.5 mm FWHM axially. The axial extension is 15 cm. The EXACT 31 system has lower spatial resolution of about 6 mm FWHM both axially and transaxially and an axial extent of about 11 cm. Most of the studies in 3D have been performed with the ECAT EXACT HR system, which is dedicated for brain studies.

In collaboration with the PET groups at the Max-Planck-Institute in Köln, Germany, at Aarhus University hospital in Denmark and at the University of California, Los Angeles, USA [Bruckbauer et al., 1995], the characteristics of the ECAT EXACT HR for 3D applications have been determined. The system was found to give 3D image data with accurate quantification. Redundancy of the data makes compression feasible. Experience from the Max-Planck-Institute in Köln indicate that the 152 Mbytes of original data may be compressed down to 11.5 Mbytes with a small degradation of the spatial resolution in the case of brain studies. At the Karolinska, the compression factor chosen leads to 23 Mbyte data sets.

The main advantage with 3D data acquisition protocols is the higher solid angle and hence the increased data collection efficiency. This higher efficiency, a factor of 4-5 relative to conventional 2D techniques, allows less smoothing to be applied during image reconstruction resulting in images with improved signal-to-noise.

ACTIVATION STUDIES

The advantage of sensitivity (and lower injected dose) has led to cerebral activation studies being performed almost exclusively in 3D. The protocols include head fixation, a transmission scan, and twelve emission scans. ^{15}O-butanol is used as the tracer since it is known to have somewhat better diffusion characteristics than water. The head fixation is used to obtain proper alignment between the transmission scan and the emission scans. Both the conventional subtraction procedures with up to three different conditions per subject and correlational approaches are currently used. The data handling is performed with a combination of the software CBA (Greitz/Bohm Computerized Brain Atlas) and the SPM package (Functional Imaging Laboratory, Wellcome Department of Cognitive Neurology, London). The procedures have been standardized to allow patient group analysis and in the past few years applied to neurological disorders such as dystonia, dyslexia, neuropathic pain, and cluster headache [Hsieh et al., 1995]. Experimental studies have been reported regarding ethanol and nicotine effects in the brain. Work is now being concentrated in the field of regulation of learning in the CNS.

RECEPTOR STUDIES

The 3D approach provides images with higher resolution and hence a better quantification in small regions. The higher efficiency in 3D results in time activity curves with less statistical noise, thus offering improved conditions for kinetic analyses of receptor ligand interaction.

PET has been extensively used to examine D1- and D2-dopamine receptors in the striatum in patients with neuropsychiatric disorders such as schizophrenia [Sedvall and Farde, 1995]. The striatum is a region of the brain with a high density of these receptor subtypes. There is increasing evidence for the involvement of extrastriatal and cortical dopaminergic systems in schizophrenia. A general problem is that the density of dopamine receptor subtypes is low in extrastriatal regions. To explore extrastriatal dopamine receptors there is thus a need for improved PET methodology.

A number of new radioligands have recently been developed. Their high affinity makes them suitable for visualization of low-density receptor populations. One example is [^{11}C]FLB 457 [Halldin et al., 1995] which has an affinity of 19 pM for D2-dopamine receptors, much higher than that of [^{11}C]raclopride with an affinity of 1000-2000 pM *in vitro*.

However, the size of the interesting regions is a potential problem. The nucleus accumbens, substantia nigra, colliculus and amygdala are considerably smaller than the striatum. Furthermore, in the neocortex, the dopamine receptors are distributed in distinct thin layers. The higher resolution and efficiency of the 3D approach is particularly suitable for examination of dopamine receptor subtypes in these small extrastriatal regions. The technique is being applied to study young, first-admission patients with schizophrenia and to identify possible target regions for antipsychotic drug treatment.

CLINICAL APPLICATIONS

In addition to the research protocols described above, 3D PET is currently applied clinically to three categories of patients. The largest cohort is a group of patients who undergo an FDG PET scan as part of an investigation for surgical treatment of epilepsy. The second group are patients being followed for recurrence after treatment for brain tumour. The use of stereotactic gamma-knife procedures for the resection of metastases has increased with the use of PET images to guide treatment planning. The improved image quality offered by 3D is particularly important in such situations where visual interpretation is part of the diagnostic process. The third group are patients referred for exploratory studies to screen the extent of malignant disease throughout the body. Whole-body studies are performed with FDG by scanning the patients in 3D at multiple bed positions.

Performing activation studies with 3D PET

UNIQUE ADVANTAGES

Widespread use is made of PET to map rCBF changes during functional brain mapping experiments, with $H_2{}^{15}O$ the most commonly used flow tracer for this application. Because of the short half-life of ^{15}O, multiple scans can be performed in each subject, separated by 8-12 minutes. Eight to eighteen flow measurements can be made during one scan session, allowing the subject to serve as his own control and to be studied under several different neuro-behavioral conditions. These experiments can take advantage of the almost linear relationship between rCBF and tissue counts with a brief "auto-radiographic" scan [Herscovitch et al., 1983]. Because the $H_2{}^{15}O$ count image closely reflects differences in quantitative rCBF, relative changes in rCBF can be determined without arterial blood sampling and the application of tracer models. This approach is now the most commonly used PET technique for functional brain mapping. Relative changes in rCBF during different tasks are determined by subtracting tissue count images that have been normalised for total brain radioactivity [Fox and Mintun, 1989; Friston et al., 1990].

The acquisition and reconstruction methods developed for 3D PET [Townsend et al., 1989] were directly applicable to these studies where relative blood flow changes are compared using qualitative images. The more challenging aspects of performing accurate normalization and attenuation and scatter correction of 3D data for full quantification did not prevent the increase in sensitivity to be used immediately. The first multi-ring BGO tomograph built with retractable septa was soon used to perform activation studies [Townsend et al., 1991].

In 3D acquisition, maximum useful count rates for a brain-sized object are obtained at close to one tenth the radioactive dose required with septa extended [Bailey et al., 1991]. Activation studies, for which up to 2 GBq doses of $H_2{}^{15}O$ are habitually administered in 2D, will exceed the optimum activity concentrations for 3D. This means that dose fractionation becomes essential, with subjects being scanned more often and with lower radiation doses than previously. Thus, more measures in each state can be obtained, or the subject scanned several times, without exceeding dose-limitation guidelines. Recent higher radiation dose estimates for $H_2{}^{15}O$ [Smith et al., 1994; Brihaye et al., 1995] have accentuated the need for high sensitivity and optimization of the dose utilization.

The gain in sensitivity offered by 3D PET has provided the ability to perform activation studies in single individuals. Small, task-specific blood flow changes from cortical areas in individual subjects can now be detected, which in the past could only be done by averaging data from groups of subjects. This has had an impact on elucidating structure-function relationships, for which purpose the PET images are combined with high resolution images of MRI. Area V5, the human visual motion area was identified in this way [Watson et al., 1993]. Data from each individual subject could be reported with more confidence than before. The individual results were superimposed on each subject's MR image in order to study the precise localization and variation in position of area V5. It proved possible in this way to identify particular landmark sulci at the occipito-temporal junction that defined the position of area V5. Thus a structure-function relationship was discovered for an area that hitherto had been considered to lie in the associated cortex.

This sensitivity gain has also enabled patients to be studied as individuals compared to normal population and permits longitudinal studies on learning and habituation effects within an individual, without exceeding radiation dose limits.

Methods developed within the context of 3D PET have enabled transient events to be detected in individuals and offers more temporal information than has hitherto been exploited. The methodology was developed to identify brain areas associated with the random, hallucinatory events experienced by schizophrenic patients. The strategy involved analysing the delivery phase of a tracer's arrival in the brain in terms of the timing and duration of activation events that occurred during that flow sensitive period. In one study, the subjects indicated, by button pressing, when experiencing hallucinations. An event-related count-rate correlational analysis [Silbersweig et al., 1994] was performed, with a score derived from the time and duration of the button pressing. Activations due to hallucinations as short as 2s have been detected with this method.

OPTIMISATION STRATEGIES

Dose fractionation. The aim in 3D PET is to fully utilise the increase in sensitivity of septaless acquisition while remaining at count rates which do not lead to excessive dead time losses for the scanner. Investigations of the noise-equivalent count (NEC) performance [Strother et al., 1990] have assessed the optimum count rate conditions that realise the maximum gain. These considerations indicate that multiple studies acquired with very small doses of $H_2{}^{15}O$ provide better signal-to-noise ratios than the equivalent dose injected as a single bolus. A factor of 3 gain in NEC was shown for 3D acquisition of $H_2{}^{15}O$ boluses of 740 MBq, relative to the 2D acquisition in a dedicated brain scanner with 10 cm axial FOV [Bailey et al., 1991]. It was also shown that by fractionating the same total dose as that administered in 2D (12 GBq total divided into 6 x 2 GBq) into a larger number of smaller doses (15 x 740 MBq), a signal-to-noise improvement in the subtraction image of a factor of 2 can be achieved compared with 2D [Cherry et al., 1993]. A recent study on a whole-body scanner with a 15 cm axial FOV has shown that more than 400 MBq in one bolus has only a limited positive effect on NECs and that dose fractionating below 100 MBq to maximize total study NECs also provides little benefit.

By increasing the number of trials per condition, dose fractionation also effectively increases the amount of time over which blood flow is being measured. This helps to average out random biological flow variations unrelated to the task. Both physical and biological arguments therefore require dose fractionation for activation studies, and especially in 3D, the former is of prime importance.

Timing of stimulus and scanning. In activation studies, the timing of stimulus presentation and scanning duration has to be optimised relative to the method of delivery of the tracer. It has been demonstrated that the rCBF distribution associated with the cognitive state is detected during the arrival of radiotracer in the brain. Slow bolus administration of the tracer [Silbersweig et al., 1993] avoids some of the timing and statistical errors and increased deadtime associated with the rapid autoradiographic bolus method while minimising the decay, CBF nonlinearity and task habituation problems associated with the longer stimulation and scanning times of the ramp infusion method. For the slow bolus (administered over 20s) this occurs over 30s and constitutes a critical temporal window during which stimulation should be performed. For these studies a scan duration of 90s was found to provide more significant activations in the areas of interest.

Data acquisition. Routine data acquisition in 3D has been limited until recently by the large data set sizes and long transfer times to memory. With the first generation of 3D PET scanners, only a small number of time frames could be acquired conveniently in 3D. In the latest generation of scanners, data averaging of the 3D data sets, both in-plane and across planes, has reduced the data set sizes considerably, and along with storage and transfer time improvements, this has enabled repeat frames of a few seconds to be acquired. For typical activation protocols, only one or two frames of data is acquired per run, and this facilitates the application of 3D PET. However, second by second total scanner count rates can be recorded and are essential in studies making use of temporal information.

Image reconstruction. The reconstruction of 3D data is mathematically more complicated than reconstruction of conventional 2D data, and requires more computation time. For activation studies with many repeated measurements, practical methods to deal with this issue had to be devised early on. With each frame taking several hours to reconstruct on workstations, a number of workstations on networks were recruited to perform the reconstruction of several activation scans in parallel. Special hardware has since been developed to reduce reconstruction times down to a few minutes (see Chapter 4). The improved statistics of 3D acquisition allows PET data sets to be reconstructed at, or close to, the resolution limit of the PET scanner, while still maintaining adequate signal to noise.

Attenuation and scatter. The method widely used for attenuation correction is based on a 2D transmission scan, acquired with septa extended, from which the 3D attenuation correction factors are generated by forward-projection (see Chapter 3). However, for activation studies, calculated attenuation is also a viable alternative.

As mentioned in previous chapters, removal of the septa increases the likelihood of detecting coincidences in which one of the gamma rays has been scattered in the head or body. The fraction of scattered events increases about threefold in 3D (see fig. 4.3) for the majority of the scanners used for activation studies. The contribution from scattered events largely cancels when images are subtracted from one another, so scatter in 3D is less concern for activation studies than it is for reconstruction of images to be used for absolute quantitation. However, the signal is contaminated. Whether this has an effect on the detection of local blood flow changes or not is still in debate. Comparisons of activation studies with and without scatter correction applied have shown little or no improvement in the significance of activated regions. Similar arguments have sometimes been used to forego normalization, attenuation and random correction in activation studies, but care must be taken when reconstructing inconsistent data.

Movement, realignment and co-registration. Performing multiple studies over scanning sessions may last several hours, and some movement of the subject is inevitable. In activation studies, the majority of this movement is likely to occur between scans during the time required to allow the isotope to decay. Accurate, automated registration techniques have been developed to deal with this problem and to realign all the PET images prior to data analysis [Woods et al., 1992]. These methods are also applied to co-register the PET images to the MR images of the same subject. Methods have also been developed to correct for the resulting mismatch of PET emission data with the transmission scan which is usually performed at the start of the study [Smith et al., 1997].

Out-of-FOV activity and shielding. Many of the latest generation of scanners are combined body and brain scanners with large apertures and axial FOVs. In these scanners, acquisition in 3D also results in a large increase in acceptance of random events originating from activity outside the FOV. These increase deadtime and hence degrade image quality. Brain scanning in particular lends itself to using additional shielding at the front of a scanner, reducing the acceptance to events originating in the body of the subject. An annular shield of thickness 9 mm positioned at the front of the gantry of the latest generation of scanners has been shown to reduce the fraction of random events acquired during an $H_2^{15}O$ scan by 50% (fig. 5.1). Over a cohort of 30 subjects, it was shown that the average NECs collected for 15 subjects scanned with the shielding was increased by 20% relative to the subjects scanned prior to the shielding being installed.

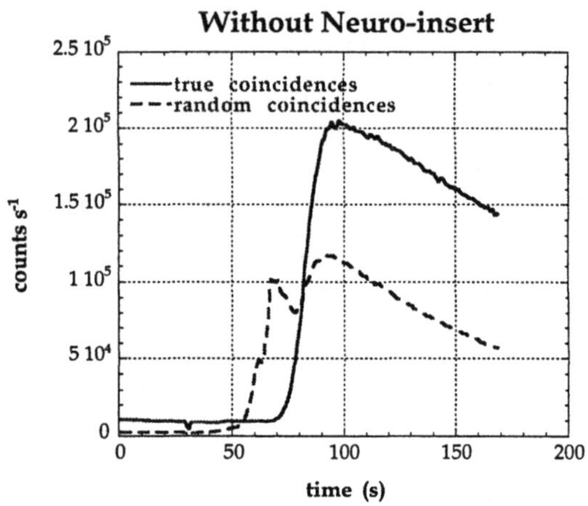

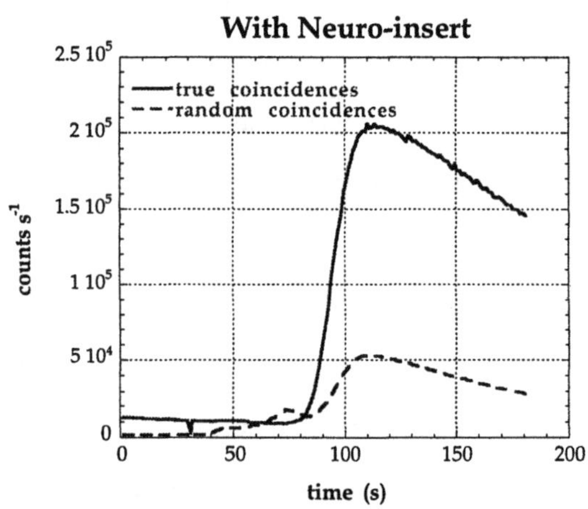

Figure 5.1 Second by second count rate data from an EXACT HR+ (solid line = total true coincidences, dashed line = random coincidences) obtained from the head of a subject scanned with (top graph) and without (lower graph) the neuro-insert in place. In both cases 37 MBq of $H_2{}^{15}O$ was infused into an antecubital vein over 20 seconds. The reduction in random coincidence rate is clearly visible both prior and during the uptake of the tracer in the brain.

Optimization of the [^{18}F]FDG protocol for clinical cerebral studies in 3D PET.

INTRODUCTION

3D PET brings the possibility of reducing both the dose injected to the patient and the acquisition duration [Cherry et al., 1991]. The reduction of the acquisition time limits the risk of patient motion and thus increases the reliability of the results. Better use can be made of the tracer by performing multiple studies from a single synthesis. The aim of this work is to evaluate and optimize the [^{18}F]FDG protocol for cerebral studies acquired in 3D PET: first, the image quality in 2D and in 3D is assessed using the noise equivalent counts (NEC) criteria [Strother et al., 1988] and second, the accuracy of both activity concentration and regional metabolism measurements in 2D and 3D modes are compared for different tracer doses.

METHOD

The study was performed on an EXACT HR+ [Brix et al., 1997]. Seven patients (5 men and 2 women) were examined in 2D and in 3D modes after an injection of [^{18}F]FDG. The injected dose was ranging from 160 to 255 MBq (4.33 to 6.9 mCi). Two-dimensional scans were acquired for 20 minutes, 30 minutes after the tracer injection. They were followed by a 5 minute scan performed in 3D. The average time between scans was 3 minutes. A headholder molded to each patient was used to maintain the head and to limit the motions during the 2D and 3D acquisitions. A 20 minute transmission scan, acquired with the septa extended, was used to compute 2D and 3D attenuation correction factors (see Chapter 3). In both modes, images were reconstructed using a Hanning window in the three directions with a 0.5/pixel cutoff frequency. The image resolution was then similar in both modes. Images were corrected for scatter using a simulation technique in 3D [Watson et al., 1995] and the 1D deconvolution in 2D [Bergström et al., 1983]. The calibration factor to convert PET counts to Bq/ml was computed in 2D and in 3D using the same calibration source (a 20 cm diameter germanium cylinder with a concentration of 4.44 kBq/ml). The reconstruction process took less than a minute in 2D and 7 minutes in 3D mode.

For each acquisition, the NEC was calculated from the total counts registered in the tomograph. The true unscattered coincidences over the field of view were derived using the scatter fraction resulting from the simulation of the scatter contribution in 3D mode [Watson et al., 1995] and the scatter fraction computed from line source measurements in 2D mode. In 3D, a value per scan was obtained, between 0.41 and 0.45, while in 2D the same value of 0.27 was used for the 7 acquisitions. The fraction of the projection bins (0.28) subtended by the head was taken into account for the computation of the number of random coincidences.

A plasma time activity curve was obtained in three patients. Images of the regional glucose metabolism were computed using three influx constants for a three compartmental model and the lumped constant [Phelps et al., 1979].

A left and right cortical ribbon of 12 mm width was defined on the radioactive concentration (CONC) images from the pixel with a value above a threshold chosen to follow the edges of the cortex. A single region-of-interest (ROI) was defined on the cerebellum using the same threshold. Circular ROIs of 1 cm diameter were also drawn on the striata and on the thalamus. This provides an average of 100 ROIs per patient.

The ROIs were reported on the corresponding cerebral glucose metabolism (CMRGlu) images. For each patient, the mean ROI value from the 2D study is plotted against the corresponding mean ROI value from the 3D study and a linear regression is applied to determine the relationship between the two sets of measurements. The slope and the correlation coefficient of the linear regression were computed with the fitted line constrained to pass through the origin. For three of the patients, the same analysis was applied to CMRGlu images.

RESULTS AND DISCUSSION

Above 200 MBq, the NEC does not increase with the injected dose (fig. 5.2) although a large variability is observed, partially due to differences between patients. To eliminate patient effects and identify the benefits associated with 3D, the ratio of the 3D NEC to 2D NEC was computed for each patient. For an injected dose ranging from 160 to 255 MBq (4.3 to 6.9 mCi) in 7 patients, an improvement in NEC greater than three (fig. 5.3), with a maximum of 3.5, is observed for 200 MBq injected dose. The scan conditions at that level of injected dose seems optimal for [^{18}F]FDG brain imaging on the EXACT HR+.

The slopes of the linear regression for the mean values of ROIs drawn on CONC images varies between 0.98 ± 0.0007 and 1.03 ± 0.007 ($p < 0.0001$ for the 7 patients) with small standard deviations (fig. 5.4). The correlation coefficients for the 7 patients are greater than 0.997. Both the slopes and the correlation coefficients indicate good agreement between 2D and 3D values.

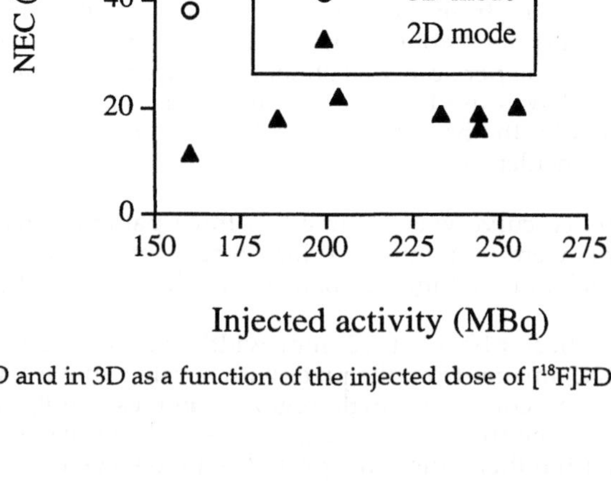

Figure 5.2 NEC in 2D and in 3D as a function of the injected dose of [^{18}F]FDG (7 patients)

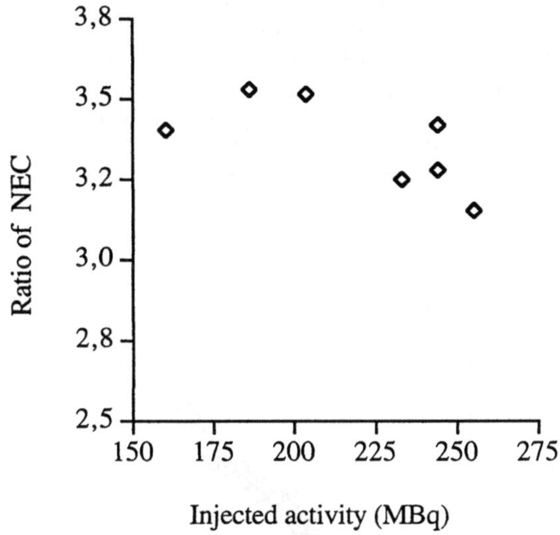

Figure 5.3 Ratio of NEC in 2D and 3D as a function of injected dose of [F^{18}]FDG (7 patients).

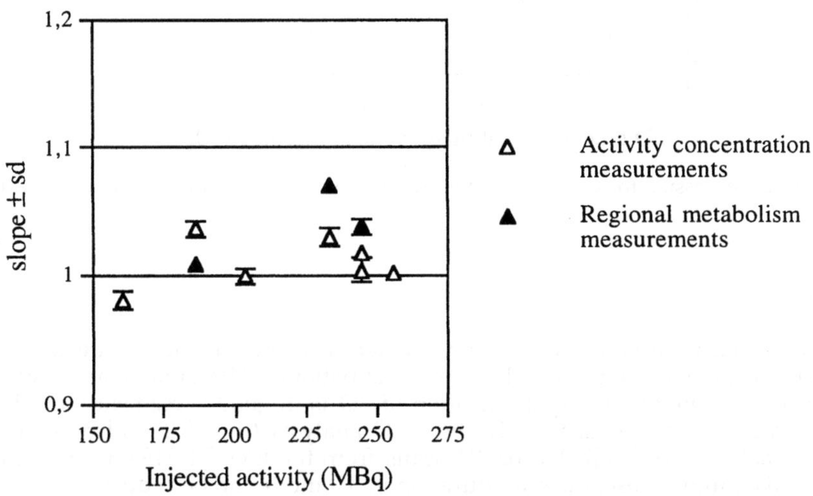

Figure 5.4 Regression slope of 3D versus 2D ROI (7 patients). Open symbols: activity concentration measurements; solid symbols: regional metabolism measurements.

Fig. 5.5 shows the linear regression of 3D versus 2D for CMRGlu measured for a patient injected with 186 MBq of [^{18}F]FDG. The slopes of the linear regression for the CMRGlu values are 1.009 ± 0.004, 1.038 ± 0.006 and 1.071 ± 0.005 ($p < 0.0001$) for the three patients. For the corresponding CONC data, the slopes are 1.036 ± 0.005, 1.004 ± 0.01 and 1.029 ± 0.007. The correlation coefficients are in good agreement with those obtained for the comparison of CONC ROI: 0.999, 0.996 and 0.947, respectively. There is a small discrepancy between the regression relationship for concentration and for metabolism that could result from the fact that the 3D scans were performed between 53 and 58 minutes post-injection, close to the period of equilibration between the tissue pool and arterial plasma; the 2D scans were acquired between 30 and 50 minutes post-injection. It has been reported that the equilibration between the tissue pool and the arterial plasma typically occurs from 60 to 100 minutes post-injection [Schmidt et al., 1996].

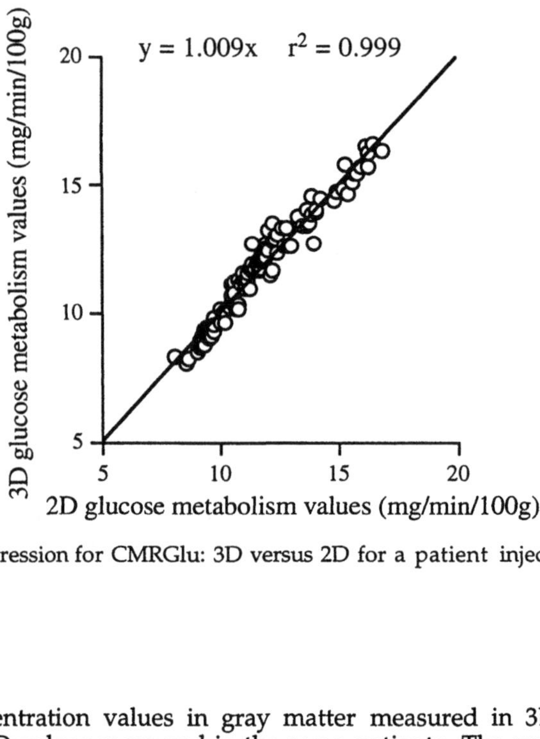

Figure 5.5 Linear regression for CMRGlu: 3D versus 2D for a patient injected with 186 MBq of FDG.

CONCLUSION.

The activity concentration values in gray matter measured in 3D mode are highly correlated to the 2D values measured in the same patients. The preliminary results for CMRGlu also illustrate that the quantification of 3D is in good agreement with the 2D values from the same patients. Clearly the NEC analysis (figs. 5.2 and 5.3) indicate that the optimal dose of [^{18}F]FDG for 3D scans from the EXACT HR+ is close to 200 MBq. With this optimal dose, the scan duration in 3D mode can be reduced by a factor of three without loss of image quality. It should also be possible to decrease the dose of [^{18}F]FDG to about 100 MBq in 3D for the same scan duration.

Contribution of 3D acquisition in pediatric neurology.

INTRODUCTION

One of the major interests of the neurological team at Louvain-la-Neuve (Belgium) concerns cerebral development [Chugani et al., 1987]. Current programs are aimed at measuring the consequences on the synaptic activity in the human brain in cases of early sensory deprivation (congenital blindness or deafness) and in children affected by neurological diseases (childhood epilepsy). To answer these questions, quantified studies of cerebral blood flow (CBF) and/or glucose metabolism (CMRGlc) are needed (preferentially both CBF and CMRGlc would be measured in a single session). Indeed, for those kind of research questions, full quantification is required because metabolic changes and the degree of synaptic density and/or activity are quantitatively related.

METHODS

As seen previously, the use of 3D acquisition allows either better resolution images to be obtained for the same radioactive dose as in 2D protocols or to lower the injected dose, which is a major advantage in clinical studies performed with children. It is well known that scatter, if not subtracted properly, reduces contrast and linearity in the images. It has been suggested that quantification would be less precise in 3D mode due to the large scatter fraction (of the order of 35% for brain). The following case study shows that this is not as dramatic as expected in the images.

In a 2D-3D comparison protocol, images were first acquired dynamically in 3D mode for 50 minutes after FDG injection (0.07 mCi/kg) in a young patient affected by epilepsy. The acquisition schedule consisted of 1 min frames from 0 to 10 minutes and 10 min frames for the next 40 minutes. Arterial blood samples were drawn for input function and glucose level determination. At the end of the scan, a 10 minute 2D frame was added for comparison purposes. Images were corrected with measured attenuation and reconstructed with and without scatter correction, using standard 2D/3D schemes available on the scanner (see Chapter 3).

RESULTS

As expected and readily apparent on fig. 5.6 and table 5.1, the scatter distribution is not stationary and the internal gray matter structures and white matter are more affected than the cortical ribbon. Nevertheless, the ratio between 3D and 2D scatter fractions is about 1.7 for all brain regions. Moreover, standard scatter correction schemes provide enough precision to obtain excellent correlation between 2D and 3D metabolic rates.

Brain region	Pixel count	SF_2D	SF_3D
frontal cortex	384	3.8%	6.5%
caudate	17	5.3%	9.1%
putamen	48	5.1%	8.7%
thalamus	34	7.0%	12.5%
white matter	25	13.3%	22.4%

Table 5.1 Scatter fraction (SF) for 2D and 3D metabolic images. The 2D and 3D images are for the same brain level in a 10 year old child studied with FDG (see text). Scatter fraction is defined as (uncorrected-corrected) / uncorrected.

As shown in table 5.2, similar metabolic rates for glucose were obtained using the autoradiographic model of Phelps [Phelps et al., 1979] and emission density data acquired in 3D or 2D modes. The use of 3D dynamic scanning in combination either with a three (3K) or four (4K) rate constant model, or with the graphical analysis of Patlak [Patlak et al.,1985] provide consistent metabolic rates at various scan periods. Only the use of the 4K model led to some overestimation of CMRGlc, due to inclusion of a k^*_4 with scan data acquired over a short time period (50 min).

Method of analysis	ARG	ARG	DYN-3K	DYN-3K	DYN-3K	DYN-4K	PATLAK
Acquisition mode	2 D	3 D	3 D	3 D	3 D	3 D	3 D
Experimental period	50' to 60'	30' to 50'	0' to 30'	0' to 40'	0' to 50'	0' to 50'	10' to 50'
Frontal cortex	53.2	55.5	54.9	54.5	53.4	58.6	50.6
Temporal cortex	48.0	49.7	50.3	49.2	48.1	53.7	45.5
Parieto-occipital cortex	46.1	47.9	50.5	48.9	47.4	55.5	44.0
Visual cortex	52.5	53.6	52.8	52.4	51.6	55.6	48.1
Striatum	47.3	50.4	51.9	49.5	47.8	56.7	44.9
Thalamus	45.3	47.9	50.6	49.1	47.2	57.2	42.9
Cerebellum	29.3	29.1	30.8	29.8	28.8	34.4	26.8
Mean cortical gray matter (right)	50.7	51.3	52.1	50.8	49.8	55.9	46.7
Mean cortical gray matter (left)	51.2	52.1	52.9	51.8	50.6	57.1	47.2

Table 5.2 Cerebral metabolic rates for glucose (CMRGlc) obtained in a 10 years old child with FDG. ARG: autoradiographic measurements of CMRGlc with rate constants: k_1=0.092 min^{-1}; k_2=0.14 min^{-1}; k_3=0.075 min^{-1}; k_4=0.0056 min^{-1}. DYN: dynamic measurements of CMRGlc using a three (3K) or four (4K) rate constants model. (LC=0.42).

DISCUSSION

Two consequences are suggested by the accuracy of 3D metabolic data. First, in the case of uncooperative patients, the higher 3D efficiency allows high-quality autoradiographic images to be obtained with accurate quantified metabolic values from a shorter total acquisition duration and, therefore, a shorter period of head restraint. A second point is that the use of lower doses allows follow-up studies in children which offers the opportunity to investigate the long-term consequences of early lesions on a longitudinal basis.

Furthermore, lowering the radioactive dose allows combined CBF-CMRGlc studies to be performed in the same child. When sufficient collaboration is obtained, repeated CBF analyses in different conditions are even possible in order to define the neural networks involved in simple physiological tasks. Activation studies in normal adult volunteers usually do not require full quantification, particularly when localization is the issue of interest. However, without full quantification it is difficult to make comparisons between individuals and a control group.

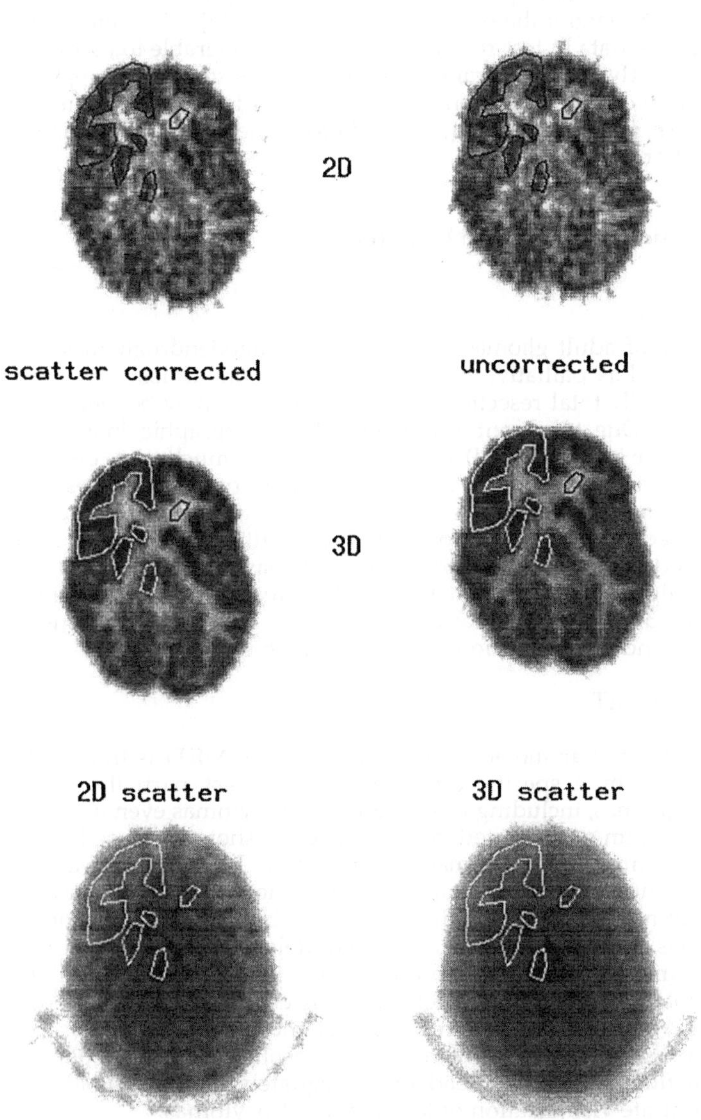

Figure 5.6 Comparison of 2D and 3D FDG images obtained at the same brain level in a 10 year old child. All images were reconstructed with a Hanning filter at 80% cutoff frequency. Upper row : 10 minute static frame, acquired in 2D, 50 minutes after tracer injection with (left) and without (right) scatter correction. Middle row: corresponding 3D images, acquired from 40 to 50 minutes after injection. Bottom row: from left to right, scatter images in 2D and 3D, respectively. For the same dose and acquisition duration, the noise reduction in the 3D images is readily apparent.

This question is especially important in a pediatric population because there are age-related changes throughout the brain [Phelps et al., 1979]. Therefore, true quantified cerebral blood flow data in test-retest conditions are preferable to investigate the neural plasticity in the early lesioned brain. The final goal is to perform repeated quantified studies, at rest and during activation, in order to investigate the coupling between blood flow and glucose metabolism. Due to radiation safety limitations this can only be achieved by 3D protocols.

Clinical applications of 3D PET in brain tumors

INTRODUCTION

To date, therapy of adult gliomas (astrocytomas, oligodendrogliomas) of grade 2 to 4 must be considered as palliative, since recurrent tumors almost invariably occur even after macroscopically total resection. Time to recurrence may be longer than 5 years in grade 2 gliomas. Due to recent improvements, tomographic imaging, in particular magnetic resonance imaging (MRI) and PET, now offers much more detailed information on tumor extent and its relation to functionally intact brain structures than previously. This opens the possibility to improve therapeutic results by applying resection, external or stereotactic radiotherapy, and application of antitumor agents in a locally precise manner, adjusted to the current stage of tumor invasiveness. It also poses a challenge to PET studies of higher brain function, to exceed the realm of cognitive science in normals and to enter the area of individual diagnostic use. This study demonstrates how 3D data acquisition and reconstruction can contribute to this goal.

C-11-METHIONINE PET

Like other large neutral amino acids, C-11-methionine (MET) is transported across the blood-brain-barrier by a specific carrier and is, at least partially, incorporated into proteins. Most gliomas, including most grade 2 astrocytomas even if they do not exhibit uptake of gadolinium or iodinated contrast agents, show increased MET uptake (i.e. more than 1.5 times the normal contralateral brain) [Ogawa et al., 1993]. Oligodendrogliomas and malignant astrocytomas show an even higher uptake (typically 2-3 times that of normal brain). Studies with serial biopsies have demonstrated that the extent of gliomas can be delineated more accurately than by CT alone [Mosskin et al., 1987]. If the tumor approaches brain structures that perform critical functions (i.e., language or motor function), exact delineation is crucial to avoid loss of that function by over extensive resection, while removing as much tumor tissue as possible. Exact delineation is possible only with low-noise high-resolution images. Poor image statistics cause random fluctuations that lead to inadequately high thresholds that may even prevent appropriate visualization of low-grade astrocytomas.

FUNCTIONAL ACTIVATION STUDIES

The gain of efficiency with 3D data acquisition permits detailed and reproducible localization of functional brain areas. In visual and somatosensory cortex, some paradigms may elicit CBF increases of more than 25%, that can be identified on individual subtraction PET images even without 3D data acquisition [Knorr et al., 1993] and on functional MRI. For most language functions, typical CBF increases are smaller. Brodmann area 22, close to the primary auditory cortex, may show typical

CBF increases in the range of 15 - 25% with simple tasks, such as repeating words [Fink et al., 1996]. More lateralized association areas, such as Broca's area, or middle and inferior temporal cortex may show CBF increases of only 5 - 15% in individual pixels, and 2 - 8 % in anatomical volumes of interest [Mazoyer et al., 1993; Herholz et al., 1996]. These signals are usually too small to be detected reliably in individuals with 2D data acquisition unless very high [O-15]water doses are applied. Even in a European multicenter study comparing the results of activation studies with stereotactic averaging across normal individuals [Poline et al., 1996], scanners with 3D data acquisition gave much more consistent and plausible results. With 3D data acquisition, i.v. bolus injection of 370 MBq for each run, and 4 replications for each condition, it has recently been shown for a verb generation task that lateralization of activation is related to hemispheric dominance and activation sites correspond with intra-operative stimulation results [Herholz et al., 1997].

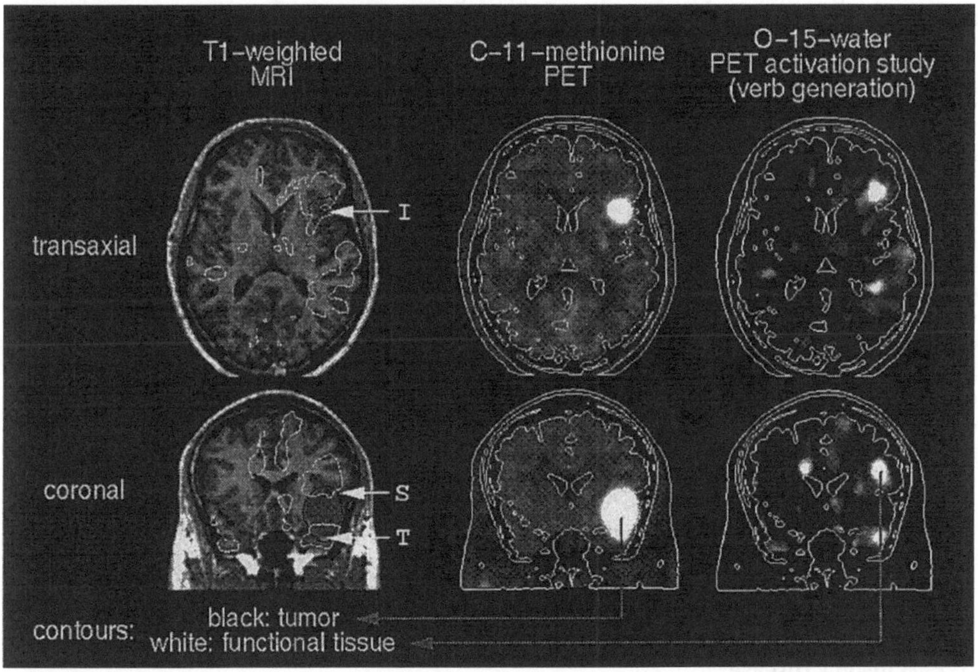

Figure 5.7 MR-, PET-methionine- and O-15-water PET activation- images of a patient with left temporal glioblastoma.

CASE REPORT

To illustrate current issues in pre-surgical diagnostics, images of a 31-year-old right-handed man, who suffered from epileptic seizures due to a left temporal glioblastoma with atypical appearance on MRI (little contrast enhancement, no edema) are shown in fig. 5.7. Although the tumor is well demarcated at the sylvian fissure (marked by "S") and its ventral border in the temporal lobe (T), the anterior border in the insula (I) is not well seen on MRI. MET PET demonstrates that most of the anterior insula is already infiltrated (black contours derived from MET PET at a level just above normal brain activity). This infiltrated area overlaps with tissue that can be functionally activated (white borders derived from activation PET at 4% CBF increase) and shows clear lateralization (patient's left is on the right of the image). Thus, the tumor does not seem to be completely resectable in this area without risk of aphasia. Some overlap of function and tumor can also be seen in the inferior temporal lobe (T). This example demonstrates that it is already possible to arrive at clinically relevant conclusions, although issues of spatial resolution and critical thresholds still require further study.

CONCLUSION

Interesting and clinically relevant issues (e.g., extent of glioma infiltration, relation to language cortex) that cannot be solved with other methods require images with very low noise and high sensitivity to detect small changes. 3D data acquisition is an important step to achieve that goal.

3D ^{18}F-Fluorodopa PET: improved kinetics and discrimination in Parkinson's disease

INTRODUCTION

Parkinson's disease is a progressive movement disorder of unknown etiology predominantly involving the nigro-striatal dopaminergic connections to the basal ganglia and is clinically characterized by poverty of movement (bradykinesia), rigidity, and a resting tremor. The main pathophysiological process is degeneration of dopaminergic neurons in the mid-brain (substantia nigra) with corresponding loss of dopaminergic nerve terminals, leading to a progressive reduction of the chemical neurotransmitter dopamine from striatal and extra-striatal regions. This has been established from post-mortem studies, which have demonstrated severe dopamine depletion in the striatum and loss of pigmented dopaminergic neurons in the substantia nigra [Bernheimer et al., 1973; Kish et al., 1988; Fearnley et al., 1991]. Consequently, it has been suggested that a 70% reduction in striatal dopamine is required before symptoms develop. Levodopa, which is a precursor of dopamine and used in the symptomatic treatment of Parkinson's disease, can be labelled with ^{18}F to produce the radiotracer ^{18}F-L-6-fluorodopa (^{18}F-fluorodopa) which in conjunction with PET scanning can be used to assess striatal pre-synaptic dopaminergic function *in vivo* [Garnett et al., 1983]. This has provided a unique opportunity to study the dopaminergic system in health and disease in "living man" and significantly contributed to our understanding of Parkinson's disease.

^{18}F-fluorodopa PET has been used to study disease degeneration and progression [Leenders et al., 1986; Vingerhoets et al., 1994a; Morrish et al., 1996], secondary Parkinsonism [Brooks et al., 1990], preclinical Parkinson's disease in at risk relatives [Burn et al., 1992], nigral dopamine cell counts [Snow et al., 1993], intracerebral fetal transplantation [Sawle et al., 1992] and striatal function in normal aging [Sawle et al., 1992; Eidelberger et al., 1993], to name a few. ^{18}F-fluorodopa PET, however, has its limitations. ^{18}F-fluorodopa is a precursor analogue of dopamine which is administered to subjects intravenously, but plasma dopa is not the primary source of endogenous brain dopa. Furthermore, ^{18}F-fluorodopa is difficult to model and quantify because of peripheral metabolism to dopa metabolites (3-O-methyl dopa) which also cross the blood brain barrier. Virtually all previous reports of PET work with ^{18}F-fluorodopa have used 2D PET data acquisition, which offers moderate sensitivity and signal-to-noise compared with 3D PET. This has made it difficult to study subregional changes within the striatum or focal extra-striatal dopaminergic changes e.g., midbrain or meso-frontal cortex, and may also explain why it has not been possible to clearly discriminate early PD patients from normals [Morrish et al., 1995].

We have implemented 3D acquisition and reconstruction of ^{18}F-fluorodopa PET [Rakshi et al., 1996], which offers a potential sensitivity increase of 3-4 fold globally in effective signal in brain studies compared with 2D acquisition [Bailey et al., 1991]. This results in improved signal-to-noise ratios with higher resolution and leads to a reduction in the partial volume effect and overall improvement in data quality. 3D PET, therefore, may provide a more precise method for monitoring subregional and focal changes in ^{18}F-fluorodopa uptake in Parkinson's disease and enhance our understanding of how striatal and extra-striatal pre-synaptic dopaminergic dysfunction develops and subsequently progresses. We have undertaken a number of studies with both 2D and 3D PET to assess the efficacy of the 3D approach.

METHODS

Data acquisition and reconstruction. The ^{18}F-fluorodopa datasets were acquired using an ECAT 953B NeuroECAT tomograph (3D studies) and an ECAT 931 whole body tomograph (2D studies) (both from CTI/Siemens PET Systems, Knoxville, TN, USA), applying protocols that have been previously documented [Rakshi et al., 1996]. Reconstructions were carried out off-line on a Sun Sparc workstation (Sun Microsystems, Mountain View, CA, USA) with dedicated vector processor (SuperCard, CSP Inc., Billerica, MA, USA) and software (LBC Inc., Knoxville, TN, USA). To test the accuracy of 3D data acquisition, reconstruction and analysis, a validation experiment simulating a patient study was performed on the ECAT 953B [Rakshi et al., 1995].

Subject data. Twelve normal subjects, mean age 57±11 years were scanned in 3D mode, including five subjects who were scanned twice (3 subjects one month apart and 2 subjects two years apart). These data were compared with data obtained from 8 different normal subjects previously scanned using a 2D protocol on the ECAT 931. Ten patients with early hemi-parkinsonism, mean age 56±8 years, mean duration of symptoms 19±5 months and mean motor Unified Parkinson's Disease Rating Scale (UPDRS) 8±3 were scanned with 3D PET. This data was compared with a previous 2D study of hemi-parkinsonism [Morrish et al., 1995]. Hemiparkinsonism is defined as patients who on motor UPDRS score have clinical signs affecting only one side of the body, e.g. in left hemi-PD, right arm and leg are normal on motor UPDRS.

Scanning protocol. All subjects were given oral doses of 150 mg of carbidopa and 400 mg of entacapone (Orion Farmos Pharmaceuticals, Espoo, Finland) one hour before scanning. A 10-minute transmission scan was performed prior to tracer injection (acquired using retractable ^{68}Ga/^{68}Ge sources). ^{18}F-fluorodopa (80 to 180 MBq) was infused intravenously over 30 seconds. The data were acquired in 3D with a protocol of 25 time frames over 94 minutes (4x1min,3x2mins,3x3mins,15x5min). The 2D data were acquired on the ECAT 931 using a protocol of 31 time frames over 94 minutes.

Data analysis. Analysis of data was performed on a Sun Sparc workstation using in-house software written in IDL (Research Systems, Inc, Boulder, CO, USA). Region of interest (ROI) analysis was performed using standardized regions of a 10 mm diameter circle ROI for head of caudate and a 10x24 mm elliptical ROI for each dorsal putamen aligned to the long axis. These regions were placed manually by visual inspection on three combined contiguous planes encompassing the striatum in 3D mode and two combined contiguous planes in 2D mode, giving equivalent total axial coverage (~18 mm). Two circular regions of 32 mm diameter were placed over the occipital lobes in the same planes as those used for the striatal regions and averaged to provide a tissue input function.

Mean counts per pixel were measured for each caudate and putamen in the last 14 frames, corresponding to the period 25-94 minutes after injection. ^{18}F-fluorodopa influx rate constants K_i^o were then calculated for each caudate and putamen using the multiple time graphical analysis method [Rutland et al., 1979; Gjedde, 1981; Patlak et al., 1983].

RESULTS

Table 5.3 demonstrates first that the mean K_i^o values for putamen and caudate were higher in 3D than in 2D mode by 29% and 21% respectively in normal subjects. Second, there was clear separation in all 10 Parkinson's disease cases of the individual symptomatic putamen K_i^o values, i.e., contralateral to the affected limb from the individual 3D normal putamen K_i^o values. The percentage reduction below the normal 3D putamen mean was 62%. All individual symptomatic putamen K_i^o values in 3D mode were more than 3 standard deviations outside the normal mean putamen K_i^o ($p<0.0001$). The mean caudate K_i^o in 3D mode contralateral to the affected limb was also significantly reduced in PD ($p<0.0001$). However, there was overlap of individual PD caudate K_i^o values with the normal caudate range. The percentage reduction below the normal caudate mean was 33%.

	3D	2D	3D
	Normals	Normals	Early hemi-PD
Sample Size	12	8	10
Putamen $K_i^o min^{-1}$	0.017 ± 0.002	0.012 ± 0.003	0.0064 ± 0.001
95% confid.interval	0.0162 to 0.0179	0.0106 to 0.0140	0.0055 to 0.0073
Range	0.0135 to 0.0209	0.0087 to 0.0169	0.0047 to 0.0091
Caudate K_i^o min^{-1}	0.016 ± 0.002	0.013 ± 0.003	0.011 ± 0.002
95% confid.interval	0.0154 to 0.0176	0.0107 to 0.0146	0.0098 to 0.0125
Range	0.0122 to 0.0233	0.0067 to 0.0182	0.0085 to 0.0146

Table 5.3 Comparison of Normal and Early PD 18F-fluorodopa data influx rate constants obtained using a reference tissue as an input function(K_i^o) in 2D and 3D PET. The K_i^o values shown for the hemiparkinsonian patients are for the putamen contralateral to the affected side.

The reproducibility in table 5.4 averages better than 5% for both the putamen and caudate, compared with the best reported reproducibility with 2D PET of approximately 10% [Vingerhoets et al., 1994b; Morrish et al., 1996]

DISCUSSION

The major putative advantage of 3D PET over 2D PET is the greater sensitivity, resulting in improved data quality. The peak count rates with equivalent administered doses of ^{18}F-fluorodopa (~130 MBq) were ~5 kcps trues in 2D on the ECAT 931 and 84 kcps trues in 3D on the ECAT 953B tomograph. The disadvantages of employing 3D ^{18}F-fluorodopa PET are the technical problems of accurate scatter correction [Trébossen et al., 1998], attenuation, detector normalization and calibration, as well as the logistical problems of larger dataset sizes and extended reconstruction times. However, the greater sensitivity permits the use of higher frequency cut-off windows in the reconstruction process to achieve higher resolution in the final images without significantly compromising the data and this, together with the increased intrinsic resolution as a consequence of smaller detector crystals in the ECAT 953B scanner, results in a reduction in the partial volume effect. This is most probably the main reason for the higher K_i^o values obtained for normals in 3D compared with 2D mode. These advantages are evident in improved image quality, more clearly defined striatal boundaries and separation of caudate from putamen. Fig. 5.8 shows a comparison of representative 5 minute time frames from ^{18}F-fluorodopa scans in different normal subjects on the four PET scanners in our Unit. The dramatic increase in image quality, in spite of decreasing administered initial doses, is clearly seen.

Subject	Putamen K_i^o (min^{-1})			Caudate K_i^o (min^{-1})		
	Scan 1	Scan 2	% Diff.	Scan 1	Scan 2	% Diff.
1	0.0185	0.0189	2	0.0175	0.0175	0
2	0.0191	0.0196	2.5	0.0177	0.0181	2
3	0.0169	0.0166	2	0.0165	0.0186	11
4	0.0146	0.0149	2	0.0145	0.0143	1
5	0.0133	0.0138	4	0.0125	0.0136	8

Table 5.4 Reproducibility of normal 3D 18F-fluorodopa data. Five subjects scanned twice to measure reproducibility showed a mean putamen variation of 2.5% and caudate variation of 4.4%. The K_i^o values are the average of left and right putamen and caudate respectively for each scan.

By using 3D ^{18}F-fluorodopa PET in 10 patients with early hemiparkinsonism, we were able to clearly discriminate in all cases, the symptomatic putamen K_i^o's from normal putamen K_i^o values. In a previous 2D study of 11 patients with early hemi-parkinsonism [Morrish et al., 1995] there was an overlap between the mean putamen Ki range in the PD group and the normal range (16 normal subjects). In a subgroup of 10 normal subjects who also had entacapone in the 2D study, the mean putamen K_i^o was 0.00121±0.003 compared with 0.0170±0.002 in our study. We conclude, therefore, that the increased sensitivity and consequently improved resolution in 3D mode allows a more precise measurement of ^{18}F-fluorodopa striatal uptake in normal subjects and hence better discrimination of patients with Parkinson's disease.

The 3D method has also demonstrated excellent reproducibility for repeated measures in the same subject, with a mean difference in K_i^o values between scans of 2.5% for putamen and 4.4% for caudate in 5 subjects. In 2D mode the documented differences reported are around 10% [Vingerhoets et al., 1994b; Morrish et al., 1996].

In conclusion, the enhanced precision and reproducibility of 3D PET allows a more accurate measurement of pre-synaptic dopaminergic function. This will allow us to detect and monitor Parkinson's disease progression more precisely, objectively assess neuroprotective therapies and study dopaminergic function in extra-striatal regions of the brain

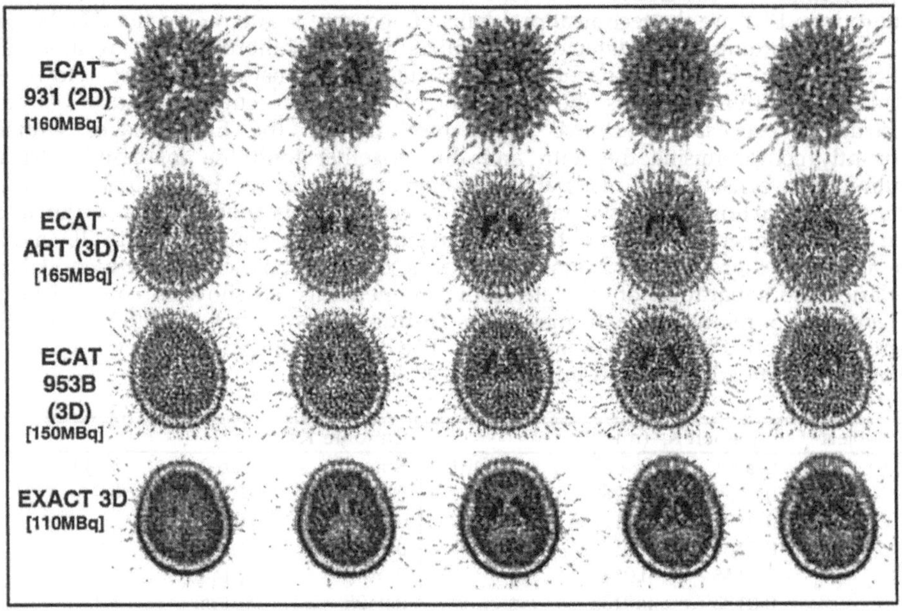

Figure 5.8 Scans from normal subjects using four different PET scanners in our Unit. All scans are 5 minute time frames taken 60 minutes after ^{18}F fluorodopa administration. The top row shows a 2D scan with our ECAT 931 [Spinks et al., 1988] whole body scanner (absolute sensitivity ~0.5%), the next row shows the ECAT ART [Bailey et al., 1997] rotating partial ring 3D tomograph (absolute sensitivity ~1.0%), the third row shows the ECAT 953B [Spinks et al., 1992] 2D/3D tomograph in 3D mode (absolute sensitivity ~3.2%), and the bottom row shows the latest generation EXACT 3D [Jones et al., 1996] whole body 3D tomograph (absolute sensitivity ~5.8%). The dose administered in each case is shown in the figure and has been decreased with increasing tomograph sensitivity.

Whole-body imaging in 3D

WHOLE-BODY IMAGING IN GENERAL TERMS

Step and shoot acquisition. Whole-body PET projection data are typically acquired in a number of axial steps of the tomograph bed in order to survey the whole patient. The number of these steps is determined by the size of the patient and the axial field-of-view (FOV) of the scanner. Whether in 2D or 3D, these segments must ultimately be combined to form an axially-long cylindrical image volume. Since the sensitivity of the scanner diminishes at its axial extremes, particularly in 3D, data acquired at adjacent bed positions must be overlapped to avoid artifacts at these seams. Increased statistical noise in these regions is the primary cause of artifacts. In both 2D and 3D modes, the bias introduced by filtered backprojection can also cause artifacts if noisy image data rather than projection data are overlapped.

Continuous axial sampling. An alternative to the step-and-shoot approach with end-to-end data assembly is to acquire the data as one long cylinder of projection data by continuously moving the patient axially through the tomograph [Dahlbom et al., 1994]. This approach is similar to that used in planar, whole-body scintigraphy. The projection data are binned with an appropriate axial offset derived from the position of the bed or the detector with respect to an initial position. Commercial PET systems do not currently possess the hardware necessary to encode this offset from a continuously moving bed. A pseudo-continuous approach in which the data are acquired in many, short-duration steps, separated by small axial increments of the bed position has been shown to improve axial uniformity and reduce normalization noise [Dahlbom et al., 1994]. These benefits must be weighed against the cost of more complex instrumentation as well as the increased patient tolerance necessary for the continuous axial motion approach.

Attenuation correction. One aspect of whole-body scanning over which there are divided opinions is the need for attenuation correction. Some investigators argue that attenuation correction makes an already long duration scan unacceptably long, with little benefit. Others would say attenuation correction is essential for quantitative results and depth-independent response. The latter is also necessary if the image volume is to be rendered for cinegraphic presentation [Wallis et al., 1990]. No comprehensive study has yet shown that lesion detection is compromised if whole-body images are interpreted without attenuation correction. The vast majority of SPECT studies are routinely interpreted this way.

If attenuation correction is used, the attenuation properties of the patient must be measured with an external source, since calculated geometric attenuation correction is inadequate in the chest. Post-injection transmission scanning [Carson et al., 1988] offers obvious logistical benefits for the long-duration scans and the consequent difficulty in achieving good emission/transmission (E/T) alignment. The time necessary to perform these measurements can be minimized with the use of image segmentation [Huang et al., 1981; Xu et al., 1991; Xu et al., 1994].

Imaging real patients. If attenuation correction is to be applied, step-and-shoot emission and post-injection transmission acquisitions are preferred for whole-body imaging to ensure E/T alignment and to allow the patient to readjust while lying in the scanner. The option to get up, walk around, and void every 30 minutes or so, without compromising the quality of the study is especially important for sick patients who may experience considerable discomfort in lying supine for an extended period of time. With these acquisition approaches, then, emission and transmission scans can be interleaved such that E and T scans are acquired sequentially and any error in repositioning the patient after a break appears as a slight axial discontinuity rather than the more severe artifacts caused by E/T misalignment.

This "interruptable" acquisition approach may not be necessary if the choice is made to forego attenuation correction. Without transmission scans, a stronger case can be made for continuous axial motion since E/T alignment is not a concern. Even for very sick oncologic patients, the total scan duration may now be tolerable for head-to-toe imaging (175 cm, 120 min), and comfortable for torso imaging (75 cm, 50 min).

3D WHOLE-BODY IMAGING

The benefits. Compared with the conventional 2D approach, true 3D collection and reconstruction of PET projection data offers the advantage in the brain of a 5-7 fold increase in the detected fraction of emitted photon-pairs being incorporated in the final image (see Chapter 4). 3D mode has been shown to yield gains in signal to noise ratio (SNR) [Cherry et al., 1992], [Dahlbom et al., 1992], [Townsend et al., 1991] or reduce patient dose while maintaining SNR. The gains are greatest at low activity since the deleterious effects of random coincidences increase rapidly with the count rate and ultimately limit the performance of the scanner without septa. The inclusion of randoms can be thought of as reducing the statistical quality of the projection data as the count-rate increases [Strother et al., 1990].

Data collection and reconstruction in 3D offers benefits not only for *in vivo* measurements of tracers with ideal imaging characteristics like ^{18}FDG, but has also helped foster investigations of new tracers with less ideal imaging characteristics. Immunoscintigraphic procedures, for example, may now be possible with PET [Cutler et al., 1995; Larson et al., 1992], whereas in 2D mode, such tracers would yield count rates inadequate for practical imaging.

The problems. 3D acquisition in the brain includes a 3-fold increase in the scatter fraction due to the elimination of septal collimation (see fig. 4.3). This can have relatively mild consequences for the quality of the data if an accurate scatter correction algorithm is used. With appropriate smoothing, the scatter distribution can be estimated and removed from the measured projections with little statistical noise added in the process. Quantitative accuracy can be restored to within a few percent, lost contrast recovered, and signal to noise maintained for a given statistical precision. In the torso, the situation is not so straightforward. Signal to noise advantages available in brain studies are all but eliminated when imaging the torso by the noisy contribution of activity outside the axial field of view (FOV). The open geometry of a long axial FOV scanner is vulnerable to random and scattered coincidences from activity just above or below the sensitive imaging volume, resulting in potentially severe degradation of image data within the axial FOV.

This effect is illustrated with a simple phantom experiment. A cylindrical scattering medium is placed in the FOV and a 0.5 mCi point source and scatter medium are placed on the tomograph axis but at various distances outside the axial FOV. These phantoms simulate a patient's torso and bladder, respectively. In 3D scanning mode, total rates of true, random and prompt coincidences are recorded with the point source positioned on the tomograph axis at 5 cm intervals from 0 to 75 cm outside the axial FOV. The resulting curves are shown in fig. 5.9.

The randoms curve starts to increase at about 35 cm indicating the beginning of the singles FOV for this tomograph. The trues curve (reflecting scattered events) rises when the point source is placed within 10 cm of the FOV, whereupon small-angle scatters are possible. The rate of random events was 3-5 times the rate of true (scattered) events throughout the measurement, indicating the relative magnitude of signal degradation from these two sources.

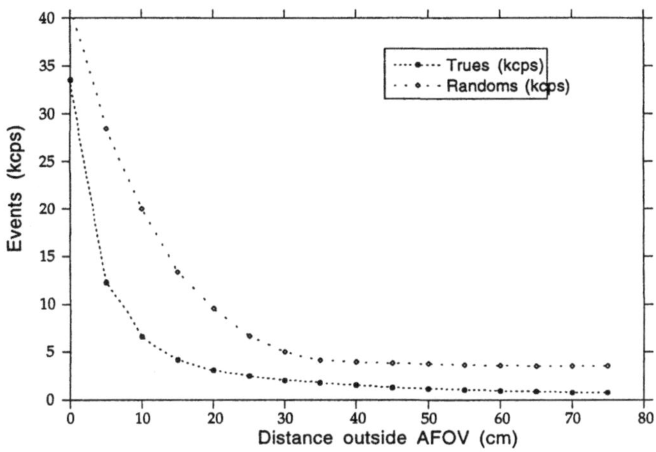

Figure 5.9 Random and scattered coincidences from a 0.5 mCi point source placed outside the axial FOV. The inflection in the randoms curve at 30-35 cm reflects the beginning of the singles FOV with the septa retracted. This corresponds to the point calculated from the gantry geometry (34 cm). The trues curve reflects scatter off a water-filled cylinder within the FOV, and rises sharply as the point source comes within 10 cm of the FOV. Signal-to-noise loss can be approximated from these curves if the count rates for activity within the FOV, and both the amount and approximate distribution of out-of-field activity are known.

For a more quantitative measurement of the signal degradation caused by out-of-field activity, a cold spot phantom can be used in place of the cylindrical scattering medium. The change in signal-to-noise can then be measured directly as the point source approaches. Fig. 5.10 shows the results of this measurement and the effects of randoms smoothing that might be used to help reduce the problem.

Obviously, out-of-field activity can not contribute useful information to the image data, so any attempt to shield the detectors from this activity will be beneficial. Additional end-shielding has been suggested and used to reduce the tomograph aperture without adversely affecting sensitivity to activity within the FOV. This approach is limited to brain applications where the neck region offers the opportunity for a reduced tomograph aperture. In imaging the torso, this approach will be less effective due to the large diameter of many patients.

Another possible solution (fig. 5.11) has been suggested [Bailey,1995] where reduced septa are used to shield detectors from out-of-field activity. While this inevitably reduces sensitivity to in-field activity, an appropriate configuration of length, thickness, and stagger would minimize this loss.

UNIQUE DIFFICULTIES WITH 3D-FILTERED BACKPROJECTION IN THE BODY

The application of multi-ring PET cameras to 3D data collection and filtered backprojection has produced a number of innovative treatments of the incomplete projection set acquired by a truncated cylindrical detector geometry. These innovations have allowed accurate backprojection over a limited set of polar angles q [Daube-Witherspoon and Muehllenher, 1987; Kinahan and Rogers, 1989; Defrise et al., 1992] without substantial cost in speed or complexity. Additional steps are necessary to form a seamless combination of the data segments of a whole-body study collected in 3D. The techniques described apply to the reprojection algorithm [Kinahan and Rogers, 1989] described in Chapter 2. The strategy in whole-body imaging is to combine axial lines of response so as to minimize the forward projection step, which is computationally-intensive, and to achieve axially uniform resolution and signal to noise. When applied sequentially to adjacent data segments of a body acquisition, this forward projection is performed redundantly along identical lines of response.

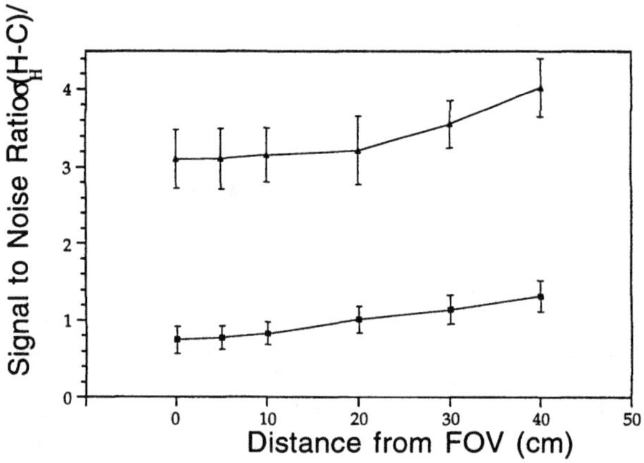

Figure 5.10 Signal-to-noise ratio in a cold spot phantom as a function of the distance of a 1 mCi point source outside the axial FOV. The signal-to-noise is degraded by almost a factor of two as the point source moves from 40 cm to the edge of the axial FOV. The upper curve represents the same data with randoms subtracted after statistical smoothing. Randoms smoothing overcomes the signal degradation from 1 mCi of out-of-field activity, and reduces the proportion of degradation caused by this activity (SNR reduction from 4.0 to 3.1 instead of 1.3 to 0.75).

Data collection. When 3D projection data are collected for a torso or whole body, each segment lacks complete 2D projections at large polar (θ) angles. These missing projections represent a collection of oblique line integrals through the patient, centered at points where adjacent bed positions meet. Forward projection to synthesize these lines of response can be eliminated entirely if adjacent bed positions are overlapped by an amount equal to the acceptance angle used in the reconstruction, designated as the maximum ring difference (Δr_{max}) in multi-ring scanners (see fig. 5.12). The obvious drawback of such an overlap is that the axial coverage for a given number of acquisition steps (bed positions) is reduced.

The choice of overlap (ov) must be made prior to acquisition of the projection data. Overlap between n bed positions must be the same for all n-1 seams in the collection, since an arbitrary spatial relationship between lines of response in each bed position would be complicated to implement during reconstruction. Absolute bed translation values, stored in the sinogram headers, are used to ensure each seam is overlapped by an integral number of detector rings, and that all overlaps are the same.

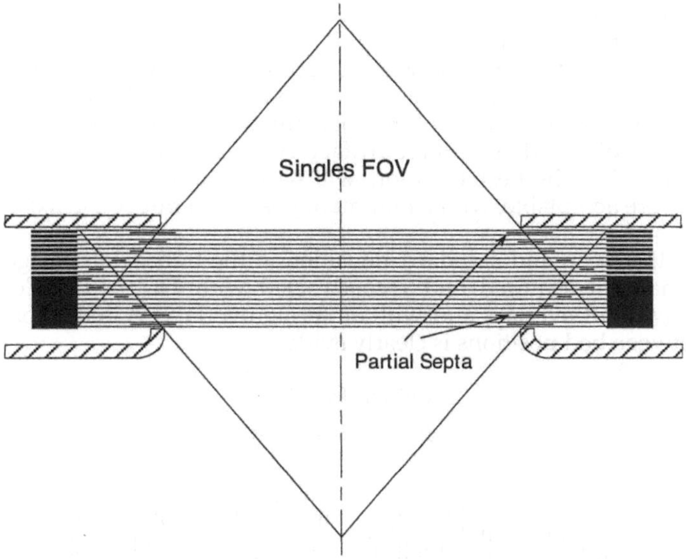

Figure 5.11 Additional end-shielding can reduce the effect of out-of-field activity, especially for brain studies, where the diameter of the patient port is not a concern, and with partial septa designed to reduce out-of-field singles, without reducing sensitivity for activity within the FOV.

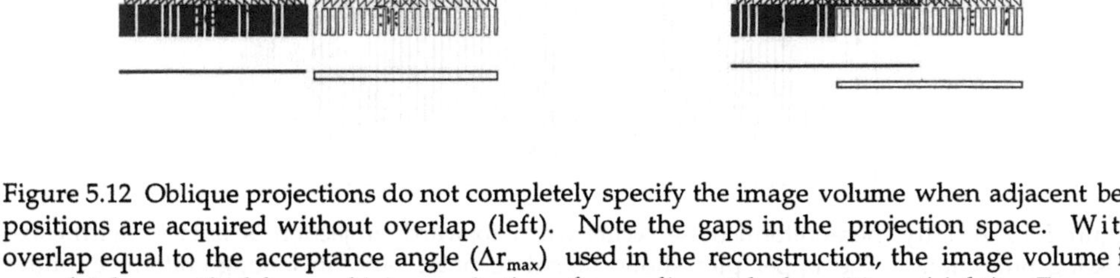

Figure 5.12 Oblique projections do not completely specify the image volume when adjacent bed positions are acquired without overlap (left). Note the gaps in the projection space. With overlap equal to the acceptance angle (Δr_{max}) used in the reconstruction, the image volume is completely specified by combining projections from adjacent bed positions (right). Forward projection is still necessary at the axial ends of the volume.

Except for the extreme ends of the volume, forward projection can be completely eliminated if the overlap matches the Δr_{max} value of the reconstruction. This configuration is undesirable because of the severe loss in axial coverage, and unnecessary since the greatest gain in reconstruction efficiency and image uniformity is obtained with the initial few rings of overlap

Reconstruction efficiency. The greatest gain in reconstruction efficiency comes from a slight overlap of just a few detector rings, for which the axial FOV is nearly unchanged, and for which a large fraction of the interpolations in the forward projection step is eliminated. Some noise and resolution artifacts may still result from the remaining forward projection, but the best trade-off will be the point at which resolution and noise uniformity are acceptable, with a minimum possible reduction in axial FOV.

Fig. 5.13 shows the mean and standard deviation in the transaxial images through a long uniform phantom acquired and reconstructed with $Dr_{max}=11$. Compared are reconstructions without overlap, and with an 8-ring overlap. A reduction in noise at the interface between bed positions is clearly evident.

Axial Uniformity

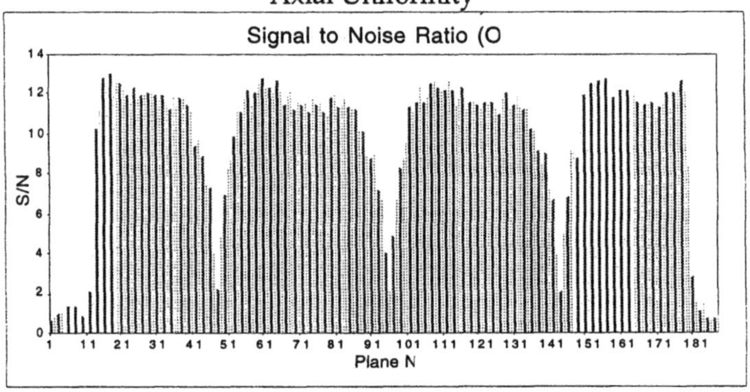

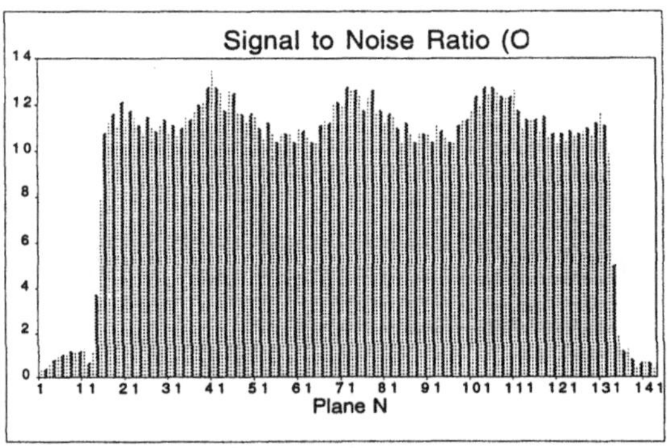

Figure 5.13 Axially non-uniform noise occurs when forward projection is used to synthesize missing projections. The upper plot shows signal to noise ratio in a long-uniform cylinder reconstructed without overlap. The lower plot shows the same parameter when the cylinder is reconstructed with an axial overlap of 8 rings. Full overlap (ov = Dr_{max}) eliminates the need for forward projection, but is unnecessary to eliminate artifacts.

Cylinder images. Fig. 5.14(a) shows coronal slices through the reconstructed uniform cylinder consisting of four bed positions with varying overlap. These images demonstrate the degree to which the axial uniformity may be improved as the overlap is increased. The four bed positions were reconstructed with the indicated overlap in detector rings and then sliced coronally to show axial modulations in mean value and variance. Note the associated reduction in the axial field-of-view. Fig. 5.14(b) shows a quantitative representation of the uniformity as measured by a large rectangular ROI centered on each coronal image. Uniformity by this measure reaches a plateau with as few as 3-4 detector rings overlapped.

(a)

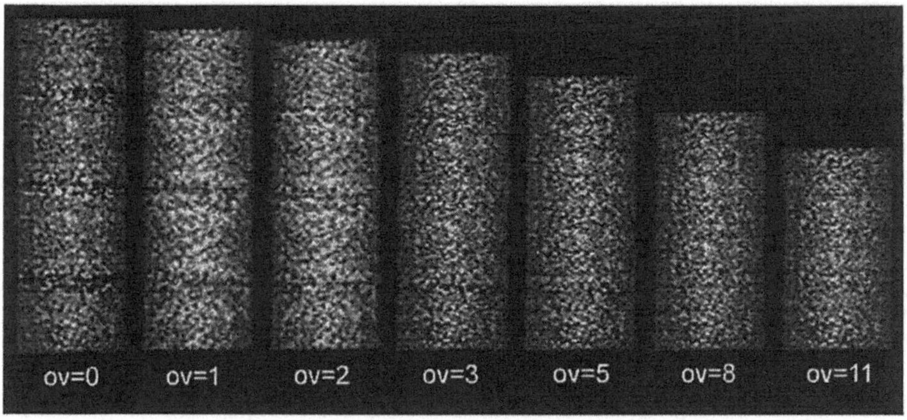

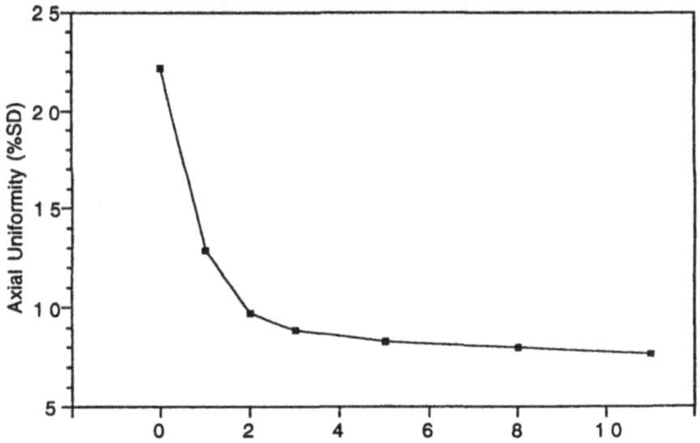

(b)

Figure 5.14 Coronal images of a long uniform cylinder reconstructed with varying overlap (a). The overlap (in detector rings) used in the reconstruction is shown. Dark bands correspond to increased noise. (b) ROI measurement of percent standard deviation in a region of interest in each coronal image are shown in the plot for various amounts of overlap used in the reconstruction.

SUMMARY

The whole body imaging approach discussed here addresses the reprojection step associated with the 3D reprojection algorithm. This proposed approach may improve resolution and noise uniformity by eliminating the reprojection step. However, these advantages must be weighed against a loss in axial coverage and potentially longer acquisition times. At most, a few rings of overlap are sufficient to smooth the transition between data segments. An overlap which eliminates the forward projection step entirely does not provide an optimum balance between uniform axial signal-to-noise and acquisition time. A simple quantitative comparison [Cutler and Xu, 1996] of the parameters affected by overlap suggests that 3 or 5 rings (depending on the scanner type) is the optimum for whole-body FDG studies.

References

Bailey DL, Jones T, Spinks TJ, Gilardi MC, and Townsend DW. Noise equivalent count measurements in a neuro-PET scanner with retractable septa. IEEE Trans Med Imag 1991;10(3):256-260.

Bailey DL. Use of partial septa for whole-body scanning. Personal Communication, 1995:

Bailey DL, Young H, Bloomfield PM, Meilke SR, Glass D, Myers MJ, Spinks TJ, Watson CC, Luk P, Peters M, Jones T. ECAT ART - a continuously rotating pet camera: performance characteristics, initial clinical studies, and installation considerations in a nuclear medicine department. Eur J Nucl Med 1997;24(1):6-15.

Bergström M, Eriksson L, Bohm C, Blomqvist G, Litton JE. Correction for scattered radiation in a ring detector positron camera by integral transformation of the projections. J Comput Assist Tomogr 1983;7(1): 42-50.

Bernheimer H, Birkmayer W, HornyKiewicz O, Jellinger K, and Seitelberger F. Brain dopamine and the syndromes of Parkinson and Huntington. Clinical, morphological and neurochemical correlations. J Neurol Sci 1973;20:415-455.

Brihaye C, Depresseux JC, Comar D. Radiation dosimetry for bolus administration of oxugen-15-water. J Nucl Med 1995;36: 651-656.

Brix G, Zaers J, Adam LE, Bellemann ME, Ostertag H, Trojan H, Haberkorm U, Doll J, Oberdorfer F, Lorenz WJ. Performance evaluation of a whole-body PET scanner using the NEMA protocol. J Nucl Med 1997;38(10):1614-1623.

Brooks DJ, Salmon EP, Mathias CJ, Quinn N, Leenders KL, Bannister R, Marsden CD, and Frackowiak RSJ. The relationship between locomotor disability, autonomic dysfunction, and the integrity of the striatal dopaminergic system in patients with multiple system atrophy, pure autonomic failure, and Parkinson's disease, studied with PET. Brain 1990;113:1539-1552.

Bruckbauer T, Wienhard K, Hanson S, Eriksson L, Blomquist G, Dahlbom M, Casey M: Evaluation of the ECAT EXACT HR with ACSII for Clinical Routine 3D Measurements. Proceedings of the IEEE Nuclear Science Symposium and Medical Imaging Conference; 1995 Oct 21-28, Conference records p1378-1382.

Burn DJ, Mark MH, Playford ED, Blank A, Blank A, Blank A, Blank A, Blank A, and Blank A. Parkinson's disease in twins studied with 18F-dopa and positron emission tomography. Neurology 1992;42:1894-1900.

Carson RE, Daube-Witherspoon ME, Green MV. A method for post-injection PET transmission measurements. J Nucl Med 1988;28:1558-1567.

Cherry SR, Dahlbom M, Hoffman EJ. 3D PET using a Conventional MultiSlice Tomograph without Septa. J Comput Assist Tomogr 1991;15(4): 655-668.

Cherry SR, Dahlbom M, Hoffman EJ. Evaluation of a 3D reconstruction algorithm for multi-slice PET scanners. Phys Med Biol 1992;37(3):779-90.

Cherry SR, Woods RP, Hoffman EJ and Mazziotta JC. Improved detection of focal cerebral blood flow changes using 3-D PET. J Cereb Blood Flow Metab 1993;13:630-638.

Chugani HT, Phelps ME, Mazziotta JC. Positron emission tomography study of human brain functional development. Ann Neurol 1987;22 : 487-97.

Cutler PD, Schwarz SW, Anderson CJ, Connett JM, Welch MJ, Philpott GW, Siegel BA. Dosimetry Of Copper-64-Labeled Monoclonal Antibody 1A3 As Determined By Pet Imaging Of the Torso. J of Nucl Med 1995;36(12):2363-2371.

Cutler PD, Xu M. Strategies to improve 3D whole-body PET image reconstruction. Phys Med and Biol 1996;41(8):1453-1467.

Dahlbom M, Yu D-C, Cherry SR, Chatziioannou A, Hoffman EJ. Methods for improving image quality in whole body PET scanning. IEEE Trans Nucl Sci 1992;39(4):1079-1083.

Dahlbom M, Cutler PD, Digby WM, Luk WK, Reed J. Characterization of sampling schemes for whole body PET imaging. IEEE Trans Nucl Sci 1994;41(4):1571-1576.

Daube-Witherspoon ME, Muehllenher G. Treatment of axial data in three-dimensional PET. J Nucl Med 1987;28(11):1717-1724.

Defrise M, Townsend D, Clack R. Favor: a fast reconstruction algorithm for volume imaging in PET. IEEE Medical Imaging Conference Record 1992;3:1919-1923.

Eidelberg D, Takikawa S, Dhawan D, Chaly T, Robeson W, Dahl R, Margouleff D, Moeller JR, Patlak SC, Fahn S. Striatal 18F-dopa uptake: absence of an aging effect. J Cereb Blood Flow Metab 1993;13:881-888.

Fearnley JM and Lees AJ. Aging and Parkinson's disease: substantia nigra regional selectivity. Brain 1991;114:2283-2301.

Fink GR, Herholz K, Wienhard K, Kessler J., Halber M., Bruckbauer T, Pietrzyk U, Heiss WD. Individual hemodynamic vs. metabolic functional anatomy of repeating words. Myers R, Cunningham V, Bailey D, Jones T, editors.Quantification of brain function using PET. San Diego: Academic Press; 1996; 79 pp:410-414.

Fox PT and Mintun MA. Noninvasive functional brain mapping by change-distribution analysis of averaged PET images of H215O tissue activity. J Nucl Med 1989;30:141-149.

Friston KJ, Frith CD, Liddle PF, Frackowiak RSJ. Comparing functional (PET) images: the assessment of significant change. J Cereb Blood Flow Metab 1990;10:458-466.

Garnett ES, Firnau G, and Nahmias C. Dopamine visualized in the basal ganglia of living man. Nature 1983;305:137-138.

Gjedde A. High and low affinity transport of D-glucose from blood to brain. J Neurochem 1981;36:1463-1471.

Halldin C, Farde L, Högberg T, Suhara T, Karlsson P, Nakashima Y, Swahn C. [11C]FLB457, a selective PET radioligand for examination of extrastriatal dopamine D2 receptors. Preparation, metabolite studies and in vivo distribution in the monkey brain using PET. J Nucl. Med. 1995;36:1275-1281.

Herholz K, Thiel A, Wienhard K, Pietrzyk U, vonStockhausen HM, Karbe H, Kessler J, Bruckbauer T, Halber M, Heiss WD. Individual functional anatomy of verb generation. Neuroimage 1996;3(3):185-94.

Herholz K, Reulen HJ, von Stockhausen HM, Thiel A, Ilmberger J, Kessler J, Eisner W, Yousry TA, Heiss WD. Preoperative activation and intraoperative stimulation of language-related areas in glioma patients. Neurosurgery 1997;41:1253-60.

Herscovitch P, Markham J and Raichle ME. Brain Blood Flow Measured with Intravenous H215O. I. Theory and Error Analysis. J Nucl Med 1983;24:782-789.

Hsieh JC, Belfrage M., Hansson P, Stone-Elander S. and Ingvar M.: Central Representation of Chronic Neuropathic Pain Studied by Positron Emission Tomography (PET). Pain 1995;63:225-236.

Huang SC, Carson R, Phelps M, Hoffman E, Schelbert H, Kuhl D. A boundary method for attenuation correction in positron emission tomography. IEEE Trans Nucl Sci 1981;22:627–637.

Jones T, Bailey DL, Bloomfield PM, Spinks TJ, Jones W, Vaigneur K, Reed J, Young J, Newport D, Moyers C, Casey ME, Nutt R. Performance Characteristics And Novel Design Aspects Of The Most Sensitive PET Camera Built For High Temporal And Spatial Resolution. J Nucl Med 1996;37(5):85P(Abstract).

Kinahan P, Rogers J. Analytic 3D image reconstruction using all detected events. IEEE Trans Nucl Sci 1989;NS-36:964-968.

Kish SJ, Shannak K, and Hornykiewicz O. Uneven pattern of dopamine loss in the striatum of patients with idiopathic Parkinson's disease. N Engl J Med 1988;318:876-880.

Knorr U, Weder B, Kleinschmidt A, Wirrwar A, Huang Y, Herzog H, Seitz RJ. Identification of task-specific rCBF changes in individual subjects: validation and application for PET. Journal of Computer Assisted Tomography 1993;17(4):517-28.

Larson SM, Pentlow KS, Volkow ND, Wolf AP, Finn RD, Lambrecht RM, Graham MC, Di Resta G, Bendriem B, Daghighian F, Yeh SDJ, Wang GJ, Cheung NV. PET scanning of iodine-124-3F8 as an approach to tumor dosimetry during treatment planning for radioimmunotherapy in a child with neuroblastoma. J Nucl Med 1992;33:2020-2023.

Leenders KL, Palmer AJ, Quinn N, Blank A, Blank A, Blank A, Blank A, and Blank A. Brain dopamine metabolism in patients with Parkinson's disease measured with positron emission tomograph. Neurol Neurosurg Psychiatry 1986;49:853-860.

Mazoyer BM, Tzourio N, Frak V, Syrota A, Murayama N, Levrier O, Salamon G, Dehaene S, Cohen L, Mehler J. The cortical representation of speech. Journal of Cognitive Neuroscience 1993;5:467-79.

Morrish PK, Sawle GV, and Brooks DJ. Clinical and [18F] dopa PET findings in early Parkinson's disease. J Neurol Neurosurg Psychiatry 1995;59:597-600.

Morrish PK, Sawle GV, and Brooks DJ. An [18F] dopa PET and clinical study of the rate of progression in Parkinson's disease. Brain 1996;119:585-591.

Mosskin M, von Holst H, Bergstrom M, Collins VP, Eriksson L, Johnstrom P, Noren G. Positron emission tomography with 11C-methionine and computed tomography of intracranial tumours compared with histopathologic examination of multiple biopsies. Acta Radiologica 1987;28(6):673-81.

Ogawa T, Shishido F, Kanno I, Inugami A, Fujita H, Murakami M, Shimosegawa E, Ito H, Hatazawa J, Okudera T, et al. Cerebral glioma: evaluation with methionine PET [see comments]. Radiology 1993;186(1):45-53.

Patlak CS, Blasberg RG, and Fenstermacher JD. Graphical evaluation of blood-to-brain transfer constants from multiple-time uptake data. J Cereb Blood Flow Metabol 1983;3(1):1-7.

Patlak C, Blasberg R. Graphical evaluation of blood-to-brain transfer constants from multiple-time uptake data.Generalizations. J Cereb Blood Flow Metab 1985; 5 : 584-90.

Phelps ME, Huang SC, Hoffman EJ, Selin C, SokoloffL, Kuhl DE. Tomographic measurement of local cerebral glucose metabolicrate in humans with [F-18]-2-fluoro-2-deoxy-D-glucose : validation of method. Ann Neurol 1979; 6: 371-388.

Poline JB, Vandenberghe R, Holmes AP, Friston KJ, Frackowiak RSJ. Reproducibility of PET activation studies - lessons from a multi-center european experiment - EU concerted action on functional imaging. Neuroimage 1996;4(1):34-54.

Rakshi J, Bailey DL, Morrish PK, and Brooks DJ. Implementation of 3D Acquisition, Reconstruction and Analysis of Dynamic Fluorodopa Studies. In: Myers R, Cunningham VJ, Bailey DL and Jones T, Quantification of Brain Function Using PET. San Diego: Academic Press, 1996;82-87.

Rutland MD. A single injection technique for subtraction of blood background in 131I-hippuran renograms. Br J Radiol 1979;52:134-137.

Sawle GV, Colebatch JG, Shah A, Brooks DJ, Marsden CD, and Frackowiak RSJ. Striatal function in normal aging: implications for Parkinson's disease. Ann Neurol 1990; 28: 799- 804.

Sawle GV, Bloomfield PM, Bjorklund A, et al. Transplantation of fetal dopamine neurons in Parkinson's disease: PET [18F]-6-L-fluorodopa studies in two patients with putaminal implants. Ann Neurol 1992;31(2):166-173.

Schmidt KC, Lucignani G, Sokoloff L. Fluorine-18-Fluorodeoxyglucose PET to determine regional cerebral glucose utilization: a re-examination. J Nucl Med 1996;37: 394-399.

Sedvall G, Farde L. Chemical brain anatomy in Schizophrenia. The Lancet 1995; 346:743-749.

Silbersweig DA, Stern E, Frith CD, Cahill C, Schnorr L, Grootoonk S, Spinks TJ, Clark J, Frackowiak RSJ, Jones T. Detection of 30s cognitive activation in single subjects with PET: A new low-dose H215O regional cerebral blood flow 3D imaging technique. J Cereb Blood Flow Metab 1993;13:617-629.

Smith AM, Bruckbauer T, Wienhard K, Pietrzyk U, Byars LG. Spatial transformation during 3D reconstruction in positron emission tomography. Eur J Nucl Med 1997;24:1413-1417.

Smith T, Tong C, Lammerstma AA, Butler KR, Schnorr L, Watson JDG, Ramsay S, Clark JC, Jones T. Dosimetry of intraveneously administered oxygen-15 labelled water in man: a model based on experimental human data from 21 subjects. Eur J Nucl Med 1994;21:1126-1134 .

Snow BJ, Tooyama I, McGeer EG, et al. Human positron emission tomographic [18F] fluorodopa studies correlate with dopamine cell counts and levels. Ann Neurol 1993;34:324-330.

Spinks TJ, Jones T, Gilardi MC, and Heather JD. Physical performance of the latest generation of commercial positron scanners. IEEE Trans Nucl Sci 1988;35(1):721-725.

Spinks TJ, Jones T, Bailey DL, Townsend DW, Grootoonk S, Bloomfield PM, Gilardi M-C, Sipe B, and Reed J. Physical performance of a positron tomograph for brain imaging with retractable septa. Phys Med Biol 1992;37(8):1637-1655.

Strother SC, Casey ME, Hoffman EJ. Measuring PET scanner sensitivity: relating countrates to image signal-to-noise-ratios using noise equivalent counts. IEEE Trans Nucl Sci 1990;37(2):783-788.

Townsend DW, Spinks TJ, Jones T, Geissbuhler A, Defrise M, Gilardi MC and Heather J. Aspects of 3D reconstruction for a multi-ring positron tomograph. Eur J Nucl Med 1989;15:741-745

Townsend DW, Defrise M, Geissbuhler A, Spinks T, Jones T. Three-dimensional reconstruction for a multi-ring positron tomograph. Prog Clini Biol Res 1991;363:139-54.

Townsend DW, Geissbuhler A, Defrise M, Hoffman EJ, Spinks TJ, Bailey DL, Gilardi MC and Jones T. Fully 3D reconstruction for a PET camera with retractable septa. IEEE Trans Med Imag 1991;10:505-512.

Trebossen R, Bendriem B, Ribeiro MJ, Fontaine A, Frouin V, Remy P. Validation of the 3D acquisition mode in PET for the quantitation of the F-18 fluoradopa uptake in the striatum. J Cereb Blood Flow Metab 1998: in press.

Vingerhoets FJ, Snow BJ, Lee CS, Schulzer M, Mak E, and Calne DB. Longitudinal fluorodopa positron emission tomographic studies of the evolution of idiopathic parkinsonism. Ann Neurol 1994;36:759-764.

Vingerhoets FJG, Snow BJ, Schulzer M, Morrison S, Ruth TJ, Holden JE, Cooper S, and Calne DB. Reproducibility of Fluorine-18-6-Fluorodopa Positron Emission Tomography in Normal Human Subjects. J Nucl Med 1994;35(1):18-24.

Wallis JW, Miller TR. Volume rendering in three-dimensional display of SPECT images. J Nucl Med 1990;31(8):1421-8.

Watson C, Newport D, Casey ME. A single scatter simulation technique for scatter correction in 3D PET. Proceedings of the 1995 International Meeting on Fully Three-dimensional Image Reconstruction in Radiology and Nuclear Medecine. Aix-les-Bains 1995.

Watson JDG, Myers R, Frackowiak RSJ, Hajnal JV, Woods RP, Mazziotta JC, Shipp S and Zeki S. Area V5 of the human brain: evidence from a combined study using PET and MRI. Cerebral Cortex 1993;3:20-26.

Woods RP, Cherry SR and Mazziotta JC. Rapid automated algorithm for aligning and reslicing PET images. J Comput Assist Tomogr 1992;16:620-633.

Xu EZ, Mullani NA, Gould KL, Anderson WL. A segmented attenuation correction for PET. J Nucl Med 1991;32(1):161-5.

Xu M, Luk WK, Cutler PD, Digby WM. Local threshold for segmented attenuation correction of PET imaging of the thorax. IEEE Trans Nucl Sci 1994;41(4):1532-1537.

MIX
Papier aus verantwortungsvollen Quellen
Paper from responsible sources
FSC® C105338

If you have any concerns about our products,
you can contact us on
ProductSafety@springernature.com

In case Publisher is established outside the EU,
the EU authorized representative is:
Springer Nature Customer Service Center GmbH
Europaplatz 3, 69115 Heidelberg, Germany

Printed by Libri Plureos GmbH
in Hamburg, Germany